The Race Against Time: Stopping the Spread of Antibiotic Resistance

Ravi

Contents

Chapter I: Introduction

1. Antibiotic resistance

Antibiotic resistance is one of the major concerns that modern medicine faces today, causing high morbidity and mortality globally and entailing huge economical costs (O'Neill, 2016; WHO, 2015).

Antibiotics interfere with vital bacterial mechanisms, however, through selective pressures, bacteria could evolve and develop resistance mechanisms to escape antibiotics action. The overuse and misuse of antibiotics, along with the reduced research and development of new antibacterial drugs, have aggravated the emergence and spread of antibiotic-resistant bacteria in the last decades (Figure 1). Thus, previously treatable bacterial infections are now life threatening due to a lack of effective antibacterial agents (Rossiter et al., 2017).

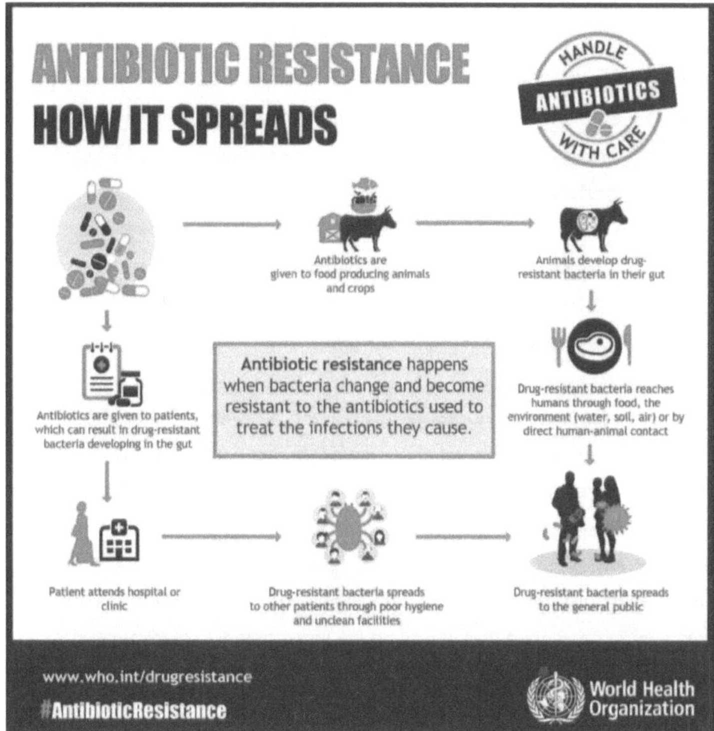

Figure 1: Antibiotic resistance emergence and spread. In a bacterial population, a few bacteria are naturally resistant to antibiotics. Antibiotic exposure in the clinic or in livestock industries results in the selection of resistant bacteria in a population that under the adequate conditions to multiply, can lead to an entire antibiotic resistant population, and can even transfer their drug resistance genes to other bacteria. Antibiotic resistance then spreads through people, livestock and other animals. Adapted from World Health organization, www.who.int/drugresistance.

The 2017 report by World Health Organization (WHO) listed the priority pathogens for the development of new antibiotics. This list is divided into three categories according to the urgency of need for new antibiotics: Critical, High and Medium priority (WHO, 2017). The three pathogens classified as Critical are:

- *Acinetobacter baumannii*, carbapenem-resistant
- *Pseudomonas aeruginosa*, carbapenem-resistant
- *Enterobacteriaceae*, carbapenem-resistant, 3rd generation cephalosporin-resistant

Six pathogens were categorized as High priority and this group includes:

- *Enterococcus faecium*, vancomycin-resistant
- *Staphylococcus aureus*, methicillin-resistant, vancomycin intermediate and resistant
- *Helicobacter pylori*, clarithromycin-resistant
- *Campylobacter*, fluoroquinolone-resistant
- *Salmonella spp.*, fluoroquinolone-resistant
- *Neisseria gonorrhoeae*, 3rd generation cephalosporin-resistant, fluoroquinolone-resistant

The least concerning group of the WHO report includes pathogens like:

- *Streptococcus pneumoniae*, penicillin-non-susceptible
- *Haemophilus influenzae*, ampicillin-resistant
- *Shigella spp.*, fluoroquinolone-resistant

Many microbes have the ability to generate secondary metabolites, specialized molecules whose production is not essential for life, but play a key role in enhancing the organism's survival and adaptation to environmental stressors. Those metabolites include a variety of compounds such as siderophores, *quorum sensing* molecules and antibiotics (Waglechner & Wright, 2017). The emergence of antibiotics as a result of secondary metabolism is believed to have happened nearly a billion years ago and that resistance must have appeared at around the same time (Waglechner & Wright, 2017). Phylogenetic analyses of methicillin-resistant *Staphylococcus aureus* (MRSA) demonstrated that the mutation that confers resistance to methicillin occurred quite before the introduction of this antibiotic in the clinic (Harkins et al., 2017). Several studies and reports converge in one idea: antibiotics and resistance are of the same age, but if before there was an equilibrium and antibiotic exposure was not sufficient for the selection and arising of resistant strains, in recent years, and mainly due to the non-therapeutic use and overuse of antibiotics generally, but specially in agriculture and livestock, microbes experienced unparalleled levels of antibiotic exposure. Consequently, bacteria have rapidly developed resistance to antibiotics and spread literally everywhere (Waglechner & Wright, 2017). It is evident that antibiotic resistance cannot be completely avoided, in fact it is a natural phenomenon, but it is fundamental to understand how resistance arises and spreads to better develop new drugs, as well as adopt behaviors to "protect" existing antibiotics and prevent the emergence and spread of further resistance mechanisms. It is of consensus that antimicrobial resistance has to be tackled in several fronts, by taking the following essential measures: (i) reduce unnecessary use of antimicrobials in agriculture and their dissemination into the environment; (ii) improve sanitation and hygiene; (iii) increase global awareness on antimicrobial resistance (AMR) among health professionals, veterinarians and general public; (iv) deploy surveillance of drug resistance and antimicrobial consumption in humans and animals; (v) promote and develop new and rapid diagnostic tools; (vi) implement stewardship (vii) invest in the development of vaccines and alternatives to antibiotics; (vii) improve funding to R&D of new antibiotics (Dodds, 2017; O'Neill, 2016; WHO, 2017).

New alternatives to traditional antibiotics to treat bacterial infections are now also being considered, such as anti-virulence agents. These drugs can, in theory, control bacterial infections not by killing the bacteria, but by affecting other pathways and mechanisms (e.g. their communication system) that reduce their virulence and ability to cause infection. Compared with traditional bactericidal approaches, inhibiting virulence is unlikely to cause the selective pressures that induce the emergence of resistance mechanisms (Rossiter et al., 2017) .

Inherent to the concept of antibiotic resistance and crucial to seek new alternatives to antibiotics, are two other fundamental concepts within this context: biofilms and *quorum sensing*, which will be approached in the next sections.

2. Bacterial biofilms and their role in antibiotic resistance

Bacteria tend to naturally accumulate and adhere to surfaces, forming sessile and sedentary communities, referred as biofilms, which can comprise many microbial species (Flemming et al., 2016).

Bacterial biofilms are defined as a population of microorganisms, in which bacterial aggregates live encased in a matrix that consists of extracellular polymeric substances (EPS) produced by the own bacteria (Linnes et al., 2013; Romaní et al., 2008; Vert et al., 2012).

Most microbial biofilms can develop attached to a surface but some aggregate in flocs, forming mobile biofilms that do not need to adhere to a surface (Flemming et al., 2016). The process of biofilm formation in a surface consists of five stages: (i) initial reversible attachment, (ii) irreversible attachment and cell-cell adhesion, (iii) proliferation, (iv) maturation and (v) dispersion (Figure 2) (Bakar et al., 2018; Jiang et al., 2020).

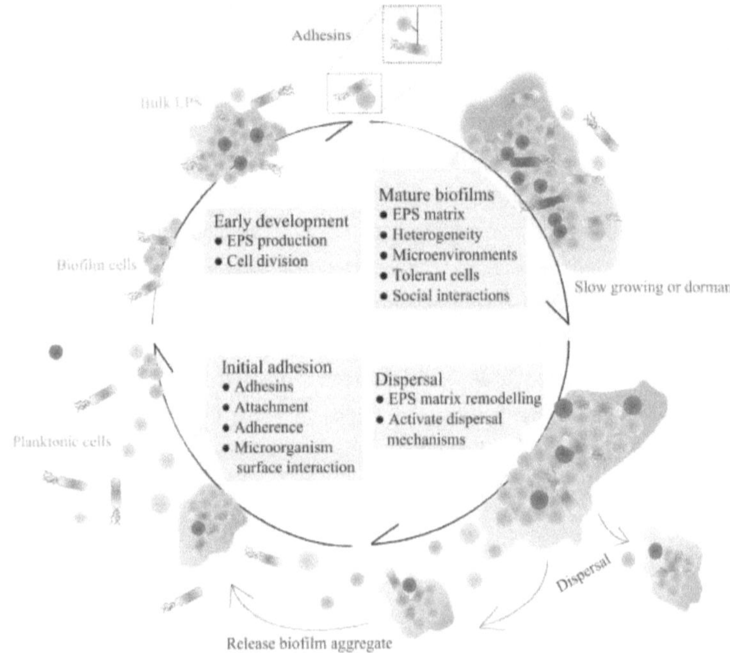

Figure 2: The five stages of biofilm development. Stage 1: Reversible attachment of free bacteria to a surface. Stage 2: Cells aggregate, forming a monolayer and producing extracellular polymeric substances (EPS), becoming irreversibly attached. Stage 3: The biofilm grows through the formation of multilayered microcolonies. Stage 4: Further growth and maturation of the biofilm, providing protection against host defense mechanisms and antibiotics. Stage 5: The biofilm disperses planktonic bacteria, ready to disseminate infection. Adapted from Jiang et al, 2020.

The starting point is the contact between free planktonic bacteria and a surface, which is still reversible at this stage. The attachment to the surface leads to the formation of a bacterial monolayer and bacteria start to produce an extracellular matrix for protection. The matrix consists of water and EPS, which include polysaccharides, structural proteins, and eDNA, as well as lipids, amyloids, cellulose, fimbriae, pili, flagellae and cell debris (Flemming & Wingender, 2010; Hobley et al., 2015; Popp & Mascher, 2019; Serra et al., 2013). These components allow the formation of channels and pores within the biofilm to facilitate the circulation of molecules (Karimi et al., 2015; Wilking et al., 2013). The matrix acts as an interface that determines the spatial architecture of the biofilm and physically bounds the biofilm system (Neu & Lawrence, 2014). The matrix is continuously remodeled and reconfigured and its formation is a dynamic process that depends essentially on environmental factors and nutrient availability, having a significative metabolic cost for the microorganism (Flemming et al., 2016; Saville et al., 2011; Whitfield et al., 2015). In the initial steps of biofilm formation, the predominant component produced is extracellular DNA (eDNA), whereas polysaccharides and structural proteins are secreted soon after. Bacteria then begin to multiply, forming microcolonies, in which the population communicate through signaling systems, such as *quorum sensing* (QS), which is often accompanied by an alteration in the bacterial growth and gene expression (Kanwar et al., 2017). As the biofilm grows and the EPS matrix starts to build up, the attachment becomes irreversible. In the last stage, some cells of the mature biofilm detach and disperse into the environment as planktonic cells to colonize and form new biofilms (Petrova & Sauer, 2016).

The biofilm self-organization is an entirely distinct lifestyle than that of planktonic cells. The structure, bacterial communication and interactions that occur within a biofilm, provide new characteristics and advantages to the microorganisms that are part of it (Stoodley et al., 2002). One unique feature of biofilms is that they allow an increased proximity between bacteria, which facilitates the formation of physical and social interactions that allow the exchange of signaling molecules and genetic material, distribution of substrate and metabolic products, and removal of toxic metabolites (Moons et al., 2009; Tielen et al., 2013; Zelezniak et al., 2015; Weipeng Zhang et al., 2015). Furthermore, the EPS matrix, along with the structure of the biofilm itself, protects the bacterial population from exposure to antibacterial agents, environmental factors, such as dehydration and shear pressure, and to the host immune system (Billings et al., 2015; Flemming & Wingender, 2010; Olsen, 2015; Weaver et al., 2015).

One of the main concerns about bacterial organization into biofilms is its reduced sensitivity to antimicrobial agents (Olsen, 2015; Yan & Bassler, 2019). The increased tolerance of biofilms to antibiotics can be explained by two major factors: (i) the properties of the molecules that compose the extracellular matrix and (ii) the slow growth rate that occurs in biofilms (Figure 3) (Balcázar et al., 2015; Flemming et al., 2016; Hathroubi et al., 2017; Li et al., 2020).

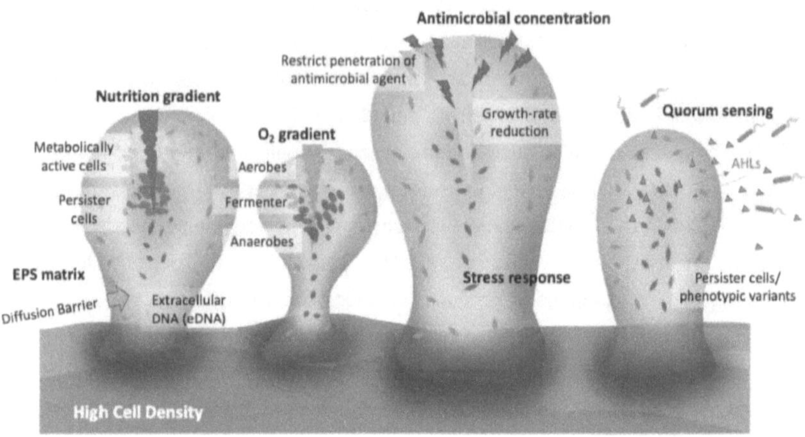

Figure 3: Factors that contribute to antimicrobial resistance in a biofilm. Nutrient and oxygen limitation leads to less metabolically active cells, which become more resistant to antibiotics than target active bacteria. Extracellular matrix acts as a protection and diffusion barrier, as well as a reservoir of enzymes that can degrade antibiotics. The high cell density and proximity of bacteria in a biofilm induce the *quorum sensing* (QS) systems, which will respond to cell density by modulating gene regulation. High cell density and increased oxidative stress observed in biofilms result in higher mutation and horizontal gene transfer rates. Adapted from Li et al, 2020.

The biofilm matrix can capture or inactivate the antimicrobial agent, representing a barrier in which the bactericidal agent cannot penetrate (Roy et al., 2018). However, some antibiotics that can get through the matrix might then be inactivated by chelation and complex formation of metallic antibiotics, enzymatic degradation or oxidizing reactions (Daddi Oubekka et al., 2012). This leads to the decrease of the concentration of the antibiotic, which by that way cannot be effective in inhibiting the bacterial growth (Zhao et al., 2020).

Moreover, the cells within the biofilm core are in stationary phase due to a concentration gradient of nutrients and oxygen (Hathroubi et al., 2017; Li et al., 2020). These cells are metabolically inactive and have a slow growth rate, called persister cells, and contribute to increased tolerance to antimicrobials that depend on the bacteria metabolism for their activity (Amato et al., 2014; Conlon et al., 2015; Maisonneuve & Gerdes, 2014).

Besides cell dormancy, resistance spread in a biofilm community can occur due to horizontal gene transfer (Mah, 2012). The high cell density and increased oxidative stress present in a biofilm leads to accumulation of eDNA and mobile genetic elements in the extracellular milieu and increases genetic competence, which enhances the uptake of resistance genes and increases mutation rate (Madsen et al., 2012; Saxena et al., 2019). Furthermore, cell density induces the coordination of virulence factors expression via QS, which allows modulation of gene expression, resulting in phenotypes that are more beneficial towards microbial endurance (Flemming & Wingender, 2010; Jiang et al., 2020). Some current strategies to inhibit or disrupt biofilm formation include targeting the EPS matrix, designing molecules that disperse the biofilm, targeting QS, and targeting dormant cells (Jiang et al., 2020).

Biofilms are particularly concerning in the clinics and in industries. Due to their reduced susceptibility to bactericidal agents, biofilms are particularly concerning in the hospital context, as they often occur in damaged tissues, as well as in medical devices, such as implants and catheters, being associated with chronic and persistent infections (Keelara et al., 2016; Olsen, 2015). Moreover, biofilms can also develop in household and industrial pipes, or biomaterials, contributing to the obstruction of tubes and filters, and corrosion of pipes (Li et al., 2020; Little & Lee, 2014), and are responsible for biofouling, contamination of process and drinking water (Mathias & Stoodley, 2011; Wingender & Flemming, 2011).

Regarding human health, biofilms can have either a negative or a positive impact. For instance, one positive aspect about biofilm formation is the protection of commensal bacterial biofilms, such as those of *Staphylococcus epidermidis*, against colonization of pathogenic bacteria, by stimulation of the immune system and prevention of adhesion (de Vos, 2015). However, biofilm development is usually associated to pathogenic conditions, being associated to various human infections, such as cystic fibrosis (CF) (Costerton et al., 1987; France et al., 2019). In CF, *Pseudomonas aeruginosa* forms biofilms in the lung epithelial cells that enable the pathogen to persist in the lung tissue, inducing a chronic CF-adapted infection for years. This is possible due to the massive production of EPS, like alginate, a matrix polysaccharide that leads to the formation of a mucoid biofilm and allows resistance to antibiotics, components of innate and adaptive immune response, and phagocytosis. Furthermore, the mucoid biofilm induces the development of a specific antibody response, which promotes chronic inflammation and indiscriminate release of oxidative species by phagocytes, resulting in further damage to the lung tissue (Bernier et al., 2013; Malhotra et al., 2019).

Due to the unique characteristics of biofilms, particularly their ability to rapidly disseminate bacteria in many diseases and decreased susceptibility to antimicrobial agents, researchers have been trying to interfere with biofilm formation, rather than inhibiting bacterial growth. Some approaches include prompting the dispersal of the biofilm or avoiding the initial formation by the development of reengineered surfaces, such as urinary catheters and implants, that block bacteria adhesion (Zhang et al., 2018).

Biofilm regulation has been extensively studied, and it has been speculated that QS may be a key factor behind antibiotic resistance associated with biofilms. Moreover, inhibiting QS could also impair biofilm formation in animal or plant tissues, medical devices and industrial surfaces, and improve the efficacy of antibacterial agents (Sankar Ganesh & Rai, 2018). Thus, QS inhibitors (QSI) have been suggested as a new strategy to overcome biofilm formation and its associated drug resistance.

3. Targeting Bacterial *Quorum Sensing* (QS)

Among the several bacterial pathways that contribute to the establishment of an infection, the QS system might be the most relevant. QS is a cell-cell communication system that coordinates several bacterial mechanisms and behaviors in a density-dependent manner, allowing bacteria to share information and modulate gene expression accordingly. QS was proved to be involved in both the formation of biofilms and the expression of virulence factors; two key mechanisms that enable bacteria to behave as pathogens, capable of colonizing and infecting/harming the host organism (Abisado et al., 2018; Bäuerle et al., 2018; Butrico & Cassat, 2020; Papenfort & Bassler, 2016; Turan et al., 2017).

This bacterial communication is achieved by the production, detection and response of small extracellular signaling molecules, known as autoinducers (AIs) that are sensed by surrounding bacteria, resulting in a response by the bacterial population such as bioluminescence, sporulation, competence, antibiotic production, biofilm formation and expression of virulence factors (production of lytic enzymes and siderophores and development of secretion systems, motility, chemotaxis and adhesion structures, etc.) (Defoirdt, 2018; Ng & Bassler, 2009). Upon production and release, these molecules accumulate in the extracellular medium as the bacterial cell density increases, and bacteria monitor and respond accordingly to the population cell number. This allows bacteria to optimize the production of virulence factors, acting in synchrony to release these molecules into the host organism only when the effect of these factors on the host will be maximized (Rutherford & Bassler, 2012).

Gram-negative and Gram-positive bacteria communicate using different QS systems, but the basic signaling mechanisms are identical. Briefly, the bacterial population produce AIs and secrete them into the extracellular medium. At high cell density, the release of this factors leads to a high concentration of AIs in the environment that is detected by cytoplasmic or membrane receptors of surrounding bacteria (Hemmati et al., 2020; Monnet & Gardan, 2015). After signal reception, these pathways act not only to activate the expression of certain genes required for pathogenesis, but also to produce and release more AIs, which may contribute to a positive regulation of these pathways to improve the communication between bacteria (Monnet & Gardan, 2015).

In Gram-negative bacteria, an AI synthase catalyzes a reaction between S-adenosylmethionine (SAM) and an acyl carrier protein (ACP) to produce an acyl homoserine lactone (AHL) (Weiwei Zhang & Li, 2016). These small molecules are detected by cytoplasmic receptors that act as transcription factors, which allows them to fold, bind DNA and regulate the expression of certain genes in the QS regulon (Figure 4A) (Banerjee & Ray, 2016; Papenfort & Bassler, 2016). This pathway also activates AI synthase expression, autoinducing signaling by AHLs (Rutherford & Bassler, 2012). In some cases of Gram-negative bacteria, AIs are detected by a histidine kinase two-component system that upon phosphorylation induces or represses expression of QS-related genes (Figure 4B) (Rutherford & Bassler, 2012).

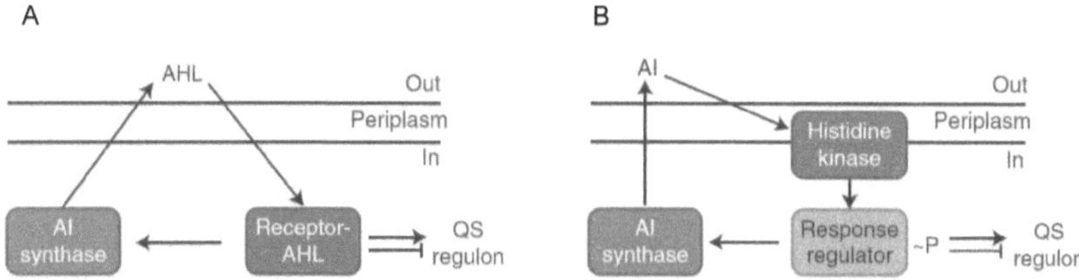

Figure 4: Bacterial *quorum sensing* (QS) systems in Gram-negative bacteria. (A) AHL small molecule QS, (B) two component signaling system. Adapted from Rutherford and Bassler, 2012.

Many Gram-positive bacteria, on the other hand, use oligopeptides, described as autoinducing peptides (AIPs). These peptides are synthetized as precursors (Pro-AIP) and processed by specialized membrane transporters that also release them into the extracellular medium (McBrayer et al., 2020; Mukherjee & Bassler, 2019). Similarly to Gram-negative bacteria, when the concentration of AIPs in the environment reaches a plateau, they bind to a membrane receptor that is part of a two-component histidine kinase signal transduction system (Boles & Horswill, 2008; Sloan et al., 2019). Once bounded, the complex is auto phosphorylated by the receptor's kinase at conserved histidines and the phosphate group is transferred to an aspartate on a cytoplasmic response regulator protein that controls gene expression of the QS regulon (Figure 5A) (Jenul & Horswill, 2019). This complex also regulates the expression of an operon that englobes the genes encoding for the pro-AIP, transporter, histidine kinase receptor and response regulator, which contributes to an autoinduction of the QS pathway (Mukherjee & Bassler, 2019). In some specific Gram-positive bacteria, the AIPs can be imported back into the cytoplasm and directly bind cytosolic transcription factors to modulate their activity (Figure 5B) (Rutherford & Bassler, 2012).

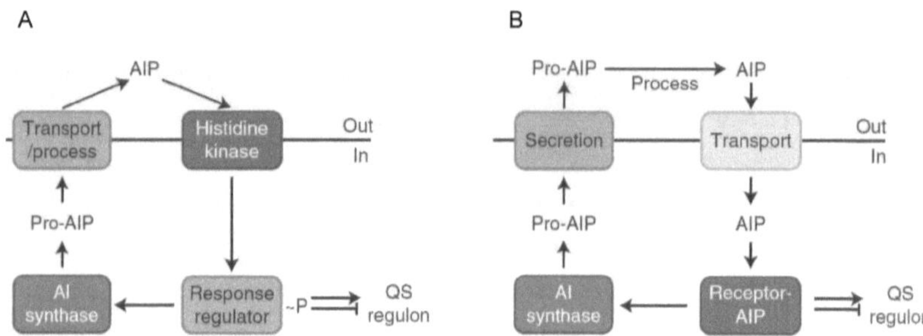

Figure 5: Bacterial *quorum sensing* (QS) systems in Gram-positive bacteria. (A) Autoinducing peptide (AIP) two-component QS, (B) AIP-binding transcription factor system. Adapted from Rutherford and Bassler, 2012.

3.1. *Pseudomonas aeruginosa Quorum Sensing*

Pseudomonas aeruginosa is a Gram-negative opportunistic pathogen that is usually found in the lungs of patients with cystic fibrosis and people who have damaged epithelial barriers, which is the case of patients who suffered severe skin burns or were submitted to tracheal or mechanical intubation, causing both acute or chronic infections (Allegretta et al., 2017; European Centre for Disease Prevention and Control, 2018). *P. aeruginosa* is naturally resistant to some conventional antibiotics, like penicillin, so the treatment for these infections rely essentially on aminoglycosides, quinolones, cephalosporins, carbapenem and polymyxins (U.S Department of Health and Human Services, 2019).

This bacterium highly depends on QS to produce virulence factors and induce infection (El-Mowafy et al., 2014). Its QS consists of four systems as follows: LasI/LasR, RhlI/RhlR, *Pseudomonas* quinolone signal (Pqs) and integrated QS signal (Iqs) (Figure 6) (Li et al., 2018; Pérez-Pérez et al., 2017; Rutherford & Bassler, 2012).

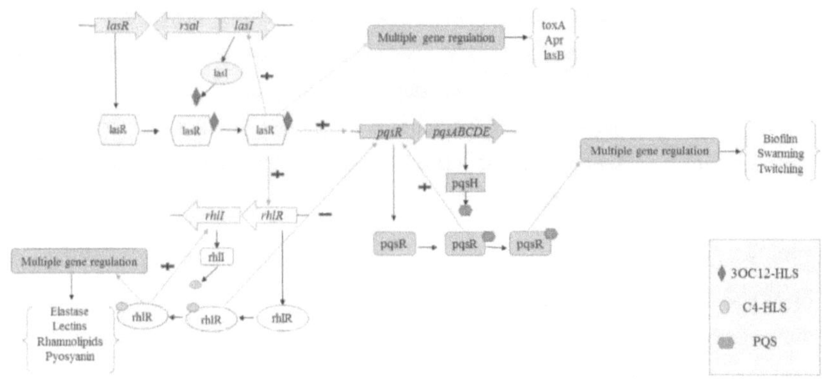

Figure 6: *P. aeruginosa* QS systems. The AHL synthases LasI, RhlI and PqsABCD produce the autoinducers 3OC12HSL, C4HSL and PQS, respectively, which are detected by the cytoplasmic transcription factors LasR, RhlR and PqsR, correspondingly. These signaling pathways regulate expression of virulence genes, as well as their corresponding AHL synthases. Adapted from Hemmati et al, 2020.

LasI synthetizes the AHL 3-oxo-C12-homoserine lactone (3OC12HSL) (Figure 6). At high AI concentration, the AHL binds to LasR and activates expression of *lasI* and virulence genes, such as those encoding elastase, protease an exotoxin A (LaSarre & Federle, 2013; Rutherford & Bassler, 2012). Furthermore, the complex LasR-3OC12HSL also induces the expression of *rhII*, that encodes for a second AI synthase, RhlI, which produces butanoyl homoserine lactone (C4HSL) (LaSarre & Federle, 2013). Upon production and secretion, this AHL binds to the cytoplasmic receptor RhlR, activating the synthesis of elastase, protease, pyocyanin and siderophores and inducing the expression of *rhII*, similarly to the LasI/LasR system (Feltner et al., 2016; LaSarre & Federle, 2013; Rutherford & Bassler, 2012).

In addition to the systems described above, the Pqs system, whose functioning mode is slightly different from the previous ones, can be mediated by 2-alkyl-quinolones (Fong et al., 2017). In this case, 2-heptyl-3-hydroxi-4-quinolone (PQS) and its biosynthetic precursor, 2-heptyl-4-hydroxyquinoline (HHQ), are synthetized by PqsABCD and PqsH and detected by the regulator PqsR (Hemmati et al., 2020). *pqsABCD* encodes proteins essential for HHQ formation, while *pqsH* encodes the last enzyme necessary for HHQ conversion to PQS (Schertzer et al., 2010).

This pathway is closely connected to the LasI/LasR and RhlI/RhlR systems, as LasR-3OC12HSL also activates the Pqs system, whereas RhlR-C4HSL represses expression of *pqsABCD* and *pqsR*. On the other hand, PqsR-PQS induces PqsABCD, resulting in further PQS and HHQ production and activation of *rhII* (LaSarre & Federle, 2013; Sun et al., 2016).

The 2-(2-hydroxyphenyl)-thiazole-4-carbaldehyde) (IQS) is a recently described signal molecule that belongs to Iqs system. It was demonstrated to integrate environmental information with the QS systems. The *ambBCDE* encodes the enzymes that lead to IQS synthesis. When IQS production is disrupted, the Pqs and Rhl systems can be disabled, interfering with the bacteria's pathogenesis (Lee et al., 2013; Lee & Zhang, 2014; Li et al., 2018).

These systems are hierarchically organized, with the LasI/LasR system at the top of the hierarchy (Defoirdt, 2018). Although it is widely assumed that QS mainly regulates the production of extracellular factors (Schuster et al., 2017), some studies have described that some intracellular components and processes can also be controlled by QS, such as the resistance to oxidative stress, phage infection and predation by protozoa in *P. aeruginosa* (Friman et al., 2013; García-Contreras et al., 2015; Moreau et al., 2017). Furthermore, the *P. aeruginosa* CRISPR-Cas system was also reported to be controlled by QS at high cell density, maximizing the bacteria immune response to phage infection (Høyland-Kroghsbo et al., 2017).

Having multiple QS systems might assure that virulence factors production occurs with optimal precision under various environmental conditions (Defoirdt, 2018). For instance, the Iqs system is able to sense nutrient limitation and partly takes over the Las system place in the QS hierarchy assuring an optimal response under environmental stress (Lee et al., 2013; Lee & Zhang, 2014; Welsh & Blackwell, 2016). Hence, a multiple subunits QS system with a dynamic hierarchy allows *P. aeruginosa* to easily adapt the QS-mediated response and establish an infection under a variety of conditions (Feltner et al., 2016; Lee & Zhang, 2014; Li et al., 2018).

When given the right conditions, these pathways lead to the production and release of a variety of virulence factors that include lectin, swarming motility, rhamnolipids, toxins and biofilm formation, in addition to those mentioned previously (Lee & Zhang, 2014). Besides, studies reported that some signal molecules, such as 3OC12HSL and PQS can also have a direct effect on the host, controlling the immune system and apoptosis of several eukaryotic cells (Liu et al., 2015). Regarding biofilm formation, it is known that it highly depends on environmental factors, however some QS regulated factors, such as rhamnolipids, swarming motility, and siderophores, also promote biofilm development in *P. aeruginosa* (Dusane et al., 2010).

As no homologous QS components have been found in humans until today, targeting these systems may be advantageous to reduce bacteria's pathogenesis, especially in persistent infections, such as those in cystic fibrosis patients (Kalia, 2013). Due to its importance in the establishment of an infection and its high position in the QS hierarchy, LasR is one of the main studied targets for anti-virulence agents, for instance, it is the target of competitive inhibitors that consist of the 3OC12HSL molecule with minor modifications (Hemmati et al., 2020; Kalia, 2013; Rossiter et al., 2017). Moreover, some LasR inhibitors have been modified to act as specific RhlR inhibitors or to antagonize both LasR and RhlR receptors (Grandclément et al., 2015; Jiang et al., 2019; Kalia, 2013). An optimal strategy would be to find compounds that can act broadly, affecting simultaneously the LasI/LasR and the RhlI/RhlR systems.

3.2. *Staphylococcus aureus Quorum Sensing*

Staphylococcus aureus is an opportunistic human pathogen that is found in the normal human skin flora, but, if given the adequate conditions, it is capable of infecting almost every organ. *S. aureus* can be responsible for causing nonthreatening infections, like minor skin infections, as well as severe diseases, such as osteomyelitis, endocarditis, necrotizing pneumonia and sepsis (Butrico & Cassat, 2020; Haaber et al., 2017). Such infections are usually treated with β-lactam antibiotics, however, as this pathogen has a great adaptive ability to overcome bactericidal agents, MRSA strains have quickly emerged. *S. aureus* became resistant to methicillin and other β-lactam antibiotics through the expression of a different PBP, the PBP2a, that is resistant to the action of methicillin and other β-lactams. MRSA isolates are often resistant to other classes of antibiotics (through different mechanisms) making treatment options limited, so the current alternatives include vancomycin, daptomycin and linezolid (Haaber et al., 2017).

PBP2a is a unique transpeptidase that is not inhibited by β-lactam antibiotics. Hence, it is able to continue peptidoglycan crosslinking in the face of the challenge by these antibiotics, when other PBPs with transpeptidase activity are inhibited.

S. aureus pathogenesis depends on the production of adhesion factors, several toxins and molecules that impact the host immune system by degrading host tissues, targeting host cells and disabling immune defenses (Butrico & Cassat, 2020; Rutherford & Bassler, 2012). Virulence and metabolic responses in *S. aureus* are controlled, partially, by QS via a two-component system encoded by the accessory gene regulator (*agr*) locus (Figure 7) (Butrico & Cassat, 2020; Jenul & Horswill, 2019).

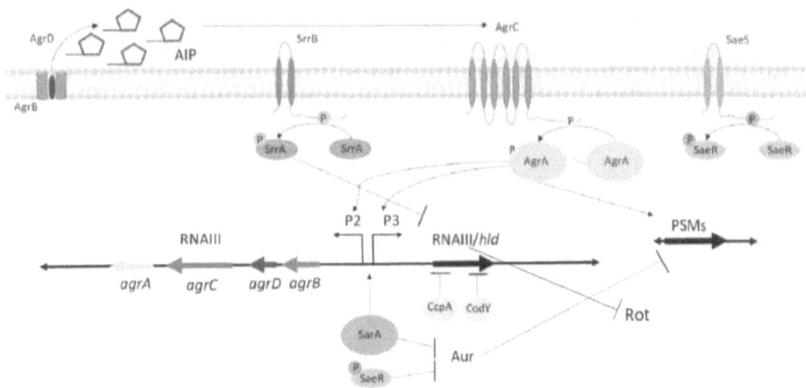

Figure 7: *S. aureus* Agr QS system. The autoinducing peptide (AIP) is synthesized in a precursor from *agrD*. AgrB processes and transports AIP to the extracellular medium. The AIP is detected by a membrane-bound histidine kinase receptor AgrC that auto phosphorylates and transfers the phosphate group to the response regulator, AgrA, which then activates the P2 and P3 promoters encoding the *agr* operon and the RNAIII regulatory RNA, respectively. RNAIII activates virulence factors production while repressing several transcription factors, such as *rot*. Some accessory regulatory proteins control virulence factor production under a variety of conditions beyond AIP concentration, including *staphylococcal* accessory regulator A (SarA), carbon catabolite control protein A (CcpA), CodY, *staphylococcal* respiratory response AB (SrrAB) and *S. aureus* exoprotein expression response regulator (SaeRS). Adapted from Butrico and Cassat, 2020.

The components Agr system are co-modulated by cross-activation of two divergent promotors, P2 and P3 (Butrico & Cassat, 2020). Briefly, P2 promoter induces expression of RNAII, whereas P3 generates RNAIII. RNAII encodes the sequences for *agrD* and *agrB*. AgrD is the pro-AIP, that is processed and secreted by the transmembrane transporter protein AgrB (Thoendel et al., 2011). On the other hand, RNAIII encodes *agrC* and *agrA* (Butrico & Cassat, 2020).

Once in the extracellular medium, the AIP binds the membrane kinase receptor AgrC, which auto phosphorylates and transfers the phosphate group to the response regulator AgrA (Boles & Horswill, 2008; Sloan et al., 2019). Like mentioned before, the phosphorylated AgrA binds the P2 promoter to autoinduce the operon and also activates the P3 promoter to initiate RNAIII expression (Rajasree et al., 2016). RNAIII activates the expression of several genes encoding virulence factors, like hemolysins, toxins and proteases, and represses the expression of surface-associated molecules involved in bacterial aggregation and adherence, including coagulase and fibronectin binding proteins A and B (Butrico & Cassat, 2020; Jenul & Horswill, 2019; Rutherford & Bassler, 2012).

Furthermore, RNAIII also represses the expression of the second immunoglobulin-binding protein (Sbi) and protein A (SpA) and increases MHC class II analog protein (Map) production (Butrico & Cassat, 2020; Chabelskaya et al., 2014; Liu et al., 2011).

RNAIII also controls the expression of transcription factors that regulate several genes. For instance, RNAIII increases the production of *mgrA*, which encodes a transcription regulator that controls more than 350 genes involved in virulence, antibiotic resistance, autolysis and biofilm formation (Gupta et al., 2015). On the other hand, RNAIII inhibits the expression of *rot*, which encodes a repressor of toxins, to induce production of additional toxins, proteases, lipases, enterotoxins, superantigens and urease (Butrico & Cassat, 2020; Rutherford & Bassler, 2012). Summarizing, in response to environmental factors, the Agr system leads to upregulation of secreted virulence factors and simultaneous downregulation of surface virulence factors, so it can go undetected by the host immune system (Hatzenbuehler & Pulling, 2011; Jenul & Horswill, 2019). Although most of the QS regulation depends on RNAIII, it has been shown that AgrA, upon phosphorylation, is also directly responsible for the production of some virulence factors, like phenol-soluble modulines (PSMs) (Butrico & Cassat, 2020). The *staphylococcal* accessory regulator (SarA) represses extracellular proteases, such as aureolysin (Aur), otherwise they would degrade PSMs (Zielinska et al., 2011).

Besides QS regulation by the *agr* locus, some additional systems have been found that allow *S. aureus* to regulate virulence factors secretion in a variety of conditions, such as oxygen concentration, oxidative stress and nutrient availability, in both Agr-dependent and independent manners. These accessory regulatory systems include SarA, CodY, catabolite control protein A (CcpA), *S. aureus* exoprotein expression (SaeRS) and *staphylococcal* respiratory response AB (SrrA/SrrB) (Cassat et al., 2013; Morrison et al., 2012; Roux et al., 2014; Rutherford & Bassler, 2012; Wilde et al., 2015).

In addition to the virulence factors mentioned above, another major weapon in the *S. aureus* virulence arsenal is biofilm development. This virulence factor is crucial for pathogenesis, as it favors resistance to antimicrobial agents. It was proved that the *agr* locus controls proteases, which affect biofilm formation *in vitro* by degrading proteins of the biofilm matrix, such as microbial surface components recognizing adhesive matrix molecules (MSCRAMMs), coagulases and PSMs (Butrico & Cassat, 2020; Cassat et al., 2013; Kolar et al., 2013; Le & Otto, 2015). However, the relevance of proteases in biofilm development *in vivo* is still unclear (Otto, 2013). It is believed that the Agr system influences biofilms *in vivo* by upregulating PSMs expression, which was proved to be involved in the structure of biofilms by forming channels and promoting cell dispersal from the biofilm to further colonize the host (Dastgheyb et al., 2015; Wang et al., 2011).

Besides, Agr-negative mutants proved to form extended biofilms, possibly due to minimal dispersal of biofilm cells resulting from low PSMs expression (He et al., 2019). Thus, on one hand, Agr is crucial for biofilm structuring and cell dissemination by PSMs expression, while disruption of Agr systems results in extended biofilm formation (Le & Otto, 2015).

Due to the rapid emergence of MRSA strains, researchers are dedicated to finding new drugs that could help treat infections caused by this pathogen. Given the importance of QS to virulence, one possible target could be the *agr* locus.

Because AIPs naturally cross-inhibit and antagonize each other, some studies have been working on developing AIP like peptides that neutralize all four types of AIPs that have been categorized to this date (Kalia, 2013; Rossiter et al., 2017).

Other studies showed the direct inhibition of AIPs by specific antibodies, reducing the production of RNAIII and toxins (Grandclément et al., 2015; Jiang et al., 2019; Kalia, 2013). However, because the *agr* system leads to biofilm disaggregation, its inhibition may lead to an improved adherence of *S. aureus* (Otto, 2004). Nevertheless, targeting the *agr* system may be a promising approach for a combinatory therapy to combat *S. aureus* and MRSA.

3.3. *Quorum Sensing* inhibitors as new anti-virulence agents

Because QS-regulated virulence factors are essential to pathogenesis, disruption of the QS systems to control or inhibit the production of such molecules appears to be an attractive strategy for the development of new drugs to treat bacterial infections. As these agents are not expected to exert selective pressures that induce drug resistance, QSI could be considered as a novel approach to treat bacterial infections by acting as anti-virulence agents (Allegretta et al., 2017). Besides, controlling the pathogen's QS-regulated virulence could reduce organization into biofilms, increasing the pathogen's sensibility to antibacterial agents and allowing the host immune system to tackle the infection more easily (Kalia, 2013; Starkey et al., 2014).

QSI can be classified as natural or synthetic compounds, or even enzymes and antibodies that act as inhibitors or antagonists on different steps of the QS pathway, such as signal molecule synthesis, detection, or transduction (Paczkowski et al., 2017; Palliyil et al., 2014; Soh et al., 2015). Some of the strategies currently in study to disrupt QS signaling include QS receptor inactivation, QS signals synthesis inhibition and degradation, and QS blockage by antibodies (Jiang et al., 2019).

Inactivation of the QS receptors is the primary approach to reduce bacterial virulence. Some compounds, such as flavonoids, N-decanoyl-L-homoserine benzyl ester and metabromo-thiolactone were proved to bind QS receptors and significantly reduce virulence factors production (O'Loughlin et al., 2013; Paczkowski et al., 2017; Weng et al., 2014; Yang et al., 2012). Besides, inhibitors of QS receptors can improve the antibacterial activity of several antibiotics, minimizing the therapeutic dose to treat infections (Capilato et al., 2017). However, these inhibitors show low stability and high degradability, and more studies are needed to improve the application of these molecules in the clinic.

In a few Gram-negative bacteria species, some AHLs proved to be able to regulate the host signaling pathways in epithelial cells and modulate immune cells behavior (Khajanchi et al., 2011; Tomioka et al., 2017). Hence, another appealing tactic to disrupt QS communication is to inhibit the synthesis of such signaling molecules. Some researchers have been able to reduce QS-regulated virulence factors production by preventing AHLs synthesis using compounds like sinefungin, S-adenosylhomocysteine and triclosan (Priyadarshi et al., 2010; Yadav et al., 2014). However, these compounds have shown a significant drawback: they also influence amino acid metabolism and interfere with bacterial vital mechanisms, which consequently leads to drug-resistance emergence by selective pressures (Copitch et al., 2010; Krol & Becker, 2014). Thus, more studies are needed to develop new inhibitors of QS signals and receptors that do not block essential nutritional metabolic pathways.

A strategy that is unlikely to cause selective pressures is the enzymatical degradation of the signal molecule once it is synthesized. For that, enzymes like AHL acylase, AHL lactonases, and oxidoreductases can be used (Grandclément et al., 2015; Hemmati et al., 2020; Jiang et al., 2020). By degrading the AI molecules, these enzymes proved to increase the bacterial susceptibility to antibacterial agents, reduce virulence factors production and inhibit biofilm formation by several important pathogens, with successful application in medical devices (Bijtenhoorn et al., 2011; Chow et al., 2014; Fan et al., 2017; Guendouze et al., 2017; Ivanova et al., 2015; Liu et al., 2016; Pustelny et al., 2009; Sakr et al., 2018). The main challenge of the use of enzymes to degrade QS AIs is their low stability in *in vivo* models, possibly due to the presence of host proteases.

Finally, some researchers have used antibodies to disrupt QS by binding to AIs, including the AHL 3OC12HSL in *P. aeruginosa*, and AIP IV in *S. aureus* (Hemmati et al., 2020; Jiang et al., 2019; Koul et al., 2016). The binding of the antibody to the AI leads to a reduction of virulence factors production and protection of the host immune cells (Hemmati et al., 2020; Jiang et al., 2019).

It is important to note that, although QSIs are not expected to induce resistance by selective pressures, point mutations that confer resistance to these agents can occur and can even be transmitted to antibiotic resistant strains. However, it is uncertain to predict if QSI-resistant strains would become dominant in a bacterial population, because it will depend on whether they would have a fitness advantage (Defoirdt et al., 2010; Mellbye & Schuster, 2011). Therefore, it is widely believed that the most effective strategy to overcome multidrug resistance will be to combine antibiotics with anti-virulence agents, specifically, QSIs. Some studies have already supported the synergistic effect of these classes of drugs. Thus, QSI reduce bacterial virulence factors production, which subsequently improves the clearance of the pathogen by the antibacterial agent, minimizing antibiotic therapeutic dosage and preventing emergence of resistant strains (Bahari et al., 2017; Christensen et al., 2012; Furiga et al., 2016; Inoue et al., 2016; Kim et al., 2018; Vadekeetil et al., 2016).

4. *Galleria mellonella* as a model organism in antimicrobial drug discovery

Mammals are commonly used by scientists as a model host species to study human and animal diseases, which is crucial for the development of novel diagnostic methods and therapies for such pathologies. However, due to cost, ethical and scientific concerns, researchers have been trying to identify alternative organisms that could be used for these studies (Andrea et al., 2019).

Among non-mammalian animal models, the larvae of the greater wax moth, *Galleria mellonella* has been extensively used to study infection and develop novel antimicrobial drugs (Freires et al., 2017).

Besides the fact that no ethical considerations are implied, *G. mellonella* can be tested at 37°C (the average body temperature) and the drug or microorganism dosage can be relatively precise (Jorjão et al., 2018). Furthermore, it shows a great correlation with results in mammals. This model presents several other advantages: high throughput screening assays at a scale that would not be possible using vertebrate models, short lifespan, convenient for handling and cost efficiency, for instance (Jønsson et al., 2017; Tsai et al., 2016).

Moreover, similarly to vertebrate animals, *G. mellonella* possess an innate immune system composed by cellular and humoral responses. The cellular response consists of rapid production of hemocytes that ingest bacteria and generate superoxide via a respiratory burst. These cells share several structural and functional comparison with mammalian phagocytes. Since phagocytes are the initial barrier to bacterial infections, *G. mellonella* larvae allow understanding of such disease processes. The humoral response includes activation of the Toll and Imd pathways that lead to activation of transcription factors, like the NF-κB family, resulting in expression of antimicrobial peptide genes (Glavis-Bloom et al., 2012; Taszłow et al., 2017; Tsai et al., 2016).

Thus, the *G. mellonella* larvae model can be used in several studies, including identification of virulence genes, drug discovery and toxicity testing (Cools et al., 2019; Fedhila et al., 2010; Silva et al., 2017).

AIMS: As mentioned above, and due to the promising application of QSI in both the clinic and the industry, this work aimed to: (i) assess the antibacterial activity of thirteen compounds and three extracts of natural/bioinspired origin against several reference strains and clinical isolates, (ii) select the compounds/extracts that did not show antibacterial activity and evaluate their capacity to impair biofilm formation in *Staphylococcus aureus* and *Pseudomonas aeruginosa* reference strains and clinical isolates using the crystal violet assay, (iii) observe the effect of extract **B** and compound **4**, which were the most effective in hampering the biofilm formation in the previous assay, in the biofilm formation by *S. aureus* and *P. aeruginosa* reference strains and multidrug-resistant (MDR) isolates by fluorescence microscopy, (iv) evaluate the effect of some of those compounds/extracts in interfering with the QS of *Chromobacterium violaceum*, through the quantification of violacein production, (v) assess the capacity of extract **B** and compound **4** to interfere with QS-related genes expression in *S. aureus* and *P. aeruginosa* reference strains and MDR isolates by quantitative reverse transcription polymerase chain reaction (RT-qPCR), (vi) assess the toxicity of **B** and **4** in the *Galleria mellonella* larvae model and (vii) evaluate the efficacy of **B** and **4** upon *G. mellonella* infection by *S. aureus*.

In parallel, another group of five compounds, obtained by chemical synthesis, were also studied as for the above points (i) and (ii) and for the potential to be photosensitizers.

Chapter II: Materials and methods

1. Organic compounds and extracts

Two groups of compounds/extracts were tested in this study and were provided by the LAQV-REQUIMTE Food Quality and Technology research group.

Group 1 included compounds designated as **0**, **1**, **2**, **3**, **4**, **5**, **8**, **10**, **11** and **14**, and extracts **A**, **B** and **C**. These compounds/extracts are of natural/bioinspired origin, being extracted from natural sources or obtained by hemisynthesis. The chemical structure of these compounds cannot be disclosed because there is a patent pending associated to them. Compound **4** is the main component of extract **A**; compound **11** is the major component of extract **B**; and compound **14** is the main component present in extract **C**.

Group 2 included compounds **15**, **16**, **17**, **18** and **19**, which were obtained by chemical synthesis and are equally associated to a process of patent pending and therefore their chemical structure cannot be revealed. These compounds are potential photosensitizers.

All compounds/extracts were provided as lyophilized powders. Stock solutions of 10 mg/mL were prepared in dimethyl sulfoxide (DMSO, Sigma-Aldrich) and stored at -20°C.

2. Bacterial strains and growth conditions

Strains used were from the American Type Culture Collection (ATCC). Clinical isolates of *Pseudomonas aeruginosa* (Pa3 and PA004) and *Staphylococcus aureus* (SA007 and SA011) were obtained from Hospital de Santo António and Hospital de São João, and were multidrug-resistant (Supplementary data, Table S1). Preceding each experiment and to obtain fresh colonies, colonies were streaked from glycerol (storage at -80°C) or milk stocks (storage at -20°C) on the respective following agar media plates. *Pseudomonas aeruginosa* ATCC 27853, *Staphylococcus aureus* ATCC 29213 and *Staphylococcus aureus* ATCC 25923, as well as Pa3, PA004, SA007 and SA011 were grown in Mueller-Hinton (MH) agar (Liofilchem srl, Italy) plates at 37°C for 24 h. *Micrococcus luteus* ATCC 4698 was grown in Tryptic Soy Broth (TSB, Liofilchem srl, Italy) supplemented with 1.5% (*w/v*) agar (Oxoid Ltd by Thermo Fisher Scientific, UK) at 30°C for 24 h. *Staphylococcus epidermidis* ATCC 14990 was grown in Nutrient Broth (NB, Liofilchem srl, Italy) supplemented with 1.5% (*w/v*) agar at 37°C for 24 h. *Streptococcus pyogenes* ATCC 19615 was grown in Brain Heart Infusion broth (BHI, Liofilchem srl, Italy) supplemented with 1.5% (*w/v*) agar and with 5% Defibrinated Sheep Blood (Thermo Fisher Scientific, USA) at 37°C with 5% CO_2 for 24 h. *Chromobacterium violaceum* ATCC 12472 was grown in Luria-Bertani (LB) medium (Liofilchem srl, Italy) supplemented with 1.5% (*w/v*) agar and incubated at 30°C for 48 h.

3. Assessing the antimicrobial activity of compounds and extracts: MIC and MBC determination

The minimum inhibitory concentration (MIC) values of all the compounds (of **Group 1** and **Group 2**) and extracts were determined by the broth microdilution method, according to the Clinical and Laboratory Standards Institute (CLSI) guidelines (Cockerill, et al, 2012). Briefly, inocula of *P. aeruginosa* ATCC 27853, *S. aureus* ATCC 29213, *M. luteus* ATCC 4698, *S. epidermidis* ATCC 14990 and *S. pyogenes* ATCC 19615 SA011 were prepared by suspending the respective fresh overnight colonies in cation-adjusted Mueller-Hinton broth (MHB2, Sigma-Aldrich, USA), which was previously supplemented with 2.5% lysed horse blood (LHB, Thermo Fisher Scientific) in the case of *S. pyogenes*, and the optical density at 600 nm (OD_{600}) was adjusted to 0.1 (corresponds to approximately 1×10^8 CFU/mL). After that, the bacterial suspension was diluted 1:100 in MHB2 to achieve 1×10^6 CFU/mL.

In a 96-well U bottom microtiter plate, 50 µL of MHB2 were dispensed from well 2 to well 12 and 100 µL of each compound/extract in a concentration 2x higher than the final that will be obtained were dispensed in well 1 and further serially diluted (two-fold dilutions) along each row. Then, 50 µL of the bacterial inoculum were added to each well, achieving a final bacterial concentration around 5×10^5 CFU/mL. For the wells containing the highest dilution, instead of the inoculum, 50 µL of MHB2 were added in order to control if the dilutions were not contaminated. Positive growth control wells contained 50 µL of MHB2 plus 50 µL of the bacterial inoculum. The negative growth control wells contained 100 µL of MHB2. A representative scheme of the inoculated microplate is shown in Figure 8, where it is also possible to see the range of concentrations tested. The microplates were incubated at 37°C for 24 h. The MIC value is defined as the lowest concentration that completely inhibits bacterial growth as detected by the naked eye. The minimum bactericidal concentration (MBC) corresponds to the lowest concentration at which no bacterial growth is observed on MH agar plates and it was determined by spreading 10 µL from the wells corresponding to / and above the MIC on MH agar plates, then incubated at 37°C for 24 h. Three independent experiments were performed.

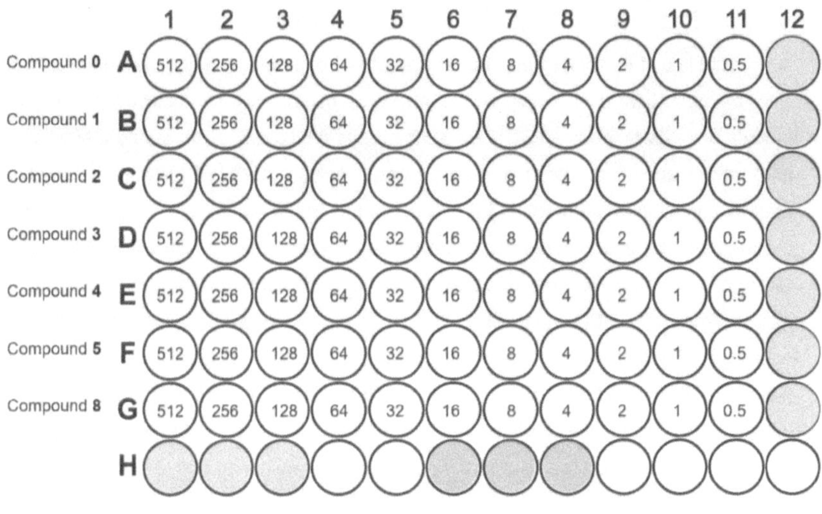

Figure 8: Exemplificative scheme of a microplate with the final concentrations of compounds or extracts (µg/mL) tested for each inoculum (e.g. *P. aeruginosa*).

4. Evaluation of biofilm formation – crystal violet assay

For the biofilm formation assay, TSB was used for *P. aeruginosa* ATCC 27853, PA004 and Pa3, whilst TSB supplemented with 1% glucose (Biochem Chemopharma, France) (TSBG) was used for *S. aureus* ATCC 29213, SA007 and SA011. All the compounds and extracts that have not shown antibacterial activity (all from **Group 1** and compounds **15**, **18** and **19** from **Group 2**), were tested at concentrations of 256, 64 and 16 µg/mL. The inocula of *P. aeruginosa* and *S. aureus* strains and isolates were prepared as above mentioned and then further diluted (1:100) in the respective medium already containing the compound or extract at the defined concentration. The samples were transferred to a flat well microplate, then incubated at 37°C for 24 h.

The planktonic phase of each well was removed, and the biofilm was washed with phosphate-buffered saline (PBS, 137 mM NaCl, 2.7 mM KCl, 10 mM Na_2HPO_4, 1.8 mM KH_2PO_4) and let air-dry. The biofilms were stained with 0.5% crystal violet (Sigma-Aldrich, USA) for 5 min, rinsed with water, air dried and resuspended in acetic acid 33% (*v/v*). The OD was measured at 595 nm. Three independent experiments were performed, each in triplicate.

5. Visualization of biofilms by fluorescence microscopy

Biofilms of *P. aeruginosa* and *S. aureus* in the presence of compound **4** or extract **B** at 64 µg/mL were observed by fluorescence microscopy after Live/Dead staining. Inocula of *P. aeruginosa* ATCC 27853, *S. aureus* ATCC 29213, Pa3, and SA011 were prepared as above mentioned and then further diluted (1:100) in the respective medium already containing the compound or extract at the concentration of 64 µg/mL, or just in the media in the case of controls. 1.5 mL of each inoculum were transferred to µ-Dish (35 mm, high), ibidi Polymer Coverslips (ibidi GmbH, Planegg-Martinsried, Germany), and biofilms were let to be formed at 37ºC for 24 h. After incubation, biofilms were rinsed once with PBS and stained using the Live/Dead staining BacLight bacterial viability kit (Molecular Probes, Thermo Fisher Scientific, MA, USA) according to the manufacturer's instructions. The stained biofilms were examined under a fluorescence microscope (widefield microscope, Zeiss Axiovert 200M), at a magnification of 630×).

6. Inhibition of *quorum sensing* in *Chromobacterium violaceum*

6.1. Qualitative assessment of QS inhibition- disc diffusion assay

The anti-*quorum sensing* activity of all the compounds (of **Group 1** and **Group 2**) and extracts was screened by the disc diffusion assay, using the violacein (purple pigment)-producing strain *C. violaceum* ATCC 12472. Colonies from a 48-h culture of *C. violaceum* ATCC 12472 were suspended in LB broth (Liofilchem srl, Italy) and the OD_{600} was adjusted to 0.1. The prepared inoculum was spread (3x) into the surface of LB agar plates, then sterile blank discs (Liofilchem srl, Italy) were placed on the top of the agar with a sterile forceps and further impregnated with 15 µL of each compound or extract at a concentration of 10 mg/mL (in DMSO). Vanillin (4-hydroxy-3-methoxybenzaldehyde, Sigma-Aldrich) at 10 mg/mL and DMSO were used as positive and negative controls, respectively. Plates were incubated at 30°C for 48 h. QS inhibition was detected by colorless, non-pigmented, colonies around the discs.

6.2. Quantitative assessment of QS inhibition - violacein pigment quantification

A few compounds and an extract from **Group 1** were selected for assessing their effects on violacein production by *C. violaceum*. The following concentrations in LB broth were tested: **B** and **4** were tested at 256, 64 and 16 µg/mL, **1** at 16 µg/mL, **2** at 64 and 16 µg/mL, **3**, **8** and **11** at 64 µg/mL. The inoculum of *C. violaceum* ATCC 12472 was prepared as above mentioned and then further diluted (1:100) in LB broth already containing the compound or extract at the defined concentration, then incubated at 30°C for 24 h. LB broth was used as a negative control and vanillin at 64 and 16 µg/mL was included as a positive control. The 24-h cultures were centrifuged at 11739 x *g* for 10 min to precipitate the insoluble violacein, the supernatant was discarded, and the pellet was resuspended in DMSO. The samples were centrifuged once more at 11739 x *g* for 10 min and the supernatant was transferred to a new microcentrifuge tube.

Afterwards, the formation of violacein by *C. violaceum* was followed by HPLC-DAD (Merck), in a reversed-phase C18 column (Agilent) with 250 × 4.6 mm i.d., particle size 2.7 µm and at 25°C. The eluents used were (i) 1% (v/v) formic acid in water and (ii) 0.5 % (v/v) formic acid in 80% (v/v) acetonitrile and the elution gradient was performed from 40 to 85% (ii) for 50 min at a flow rate of 0.4 mL/ min. After 50 min, the column was washed with 100% (ii) for 10 min and then it was stabilized with the initial conditions for more 10 min. The percentage of violacein inhibition was calculated as follows:

$$\% \text{ of violacein production inhibition} = \frac{\text{Peak area (LB control)} - \text{Peak area (treated)}}{\text{Peak area (LB control)}} \times 100$$

Two independent experiments were performed, each allowing triplicate measurements for each condition assayed.

7. Biofilm formation for RNA extraction

7.1. Biofilm formation of *P. aeruginosa* and *S. aureus* reference strains and MDR isolates

To assess the expression of *P. aeruginosa* and *S. aureus* QS-related genes, biofilms of both ATCC strains as well as of Pa3, SA007 and SA011 were formed in the absence (controls) and presence of compound **4** or extract **B** at 64 µg/mL. The inocula were prepared as above mentioned and then further diluted (1:100) in the respective medium already containing the compound or extract at the defined concentration. Each of the prepared inocula were dispensed into 6 well plates (2 mL/well), and each condition in two to four wells, and incubated at 37°C for 24 h.

Then, the planktonic phase of each well was removed, and the biofilm was washed once with PBS. The biofilm was then collected in 750 µL PBS (from one well in the case of controls, and from 3 to 4 wells in the case of biofilms formed in the presence of **B** or **4**), and using cell scrapers, to RNase/DNase free microcentrifuge tubes. The samples were centrifuged at 9030 x *g* for 2 min, the supernatant was discarded, and the pellet was resuspended in 750 µL RNA*later* (Sigma-Aldrich, USA) and stored overnight at 4°C and then at -20°C until later RNA extraction.

7.2. RNA extraction and purification

Biofilm samples stored in RNA*later* were centrifuged at 9030 x *g* for 2 min, the supernatant was discarded to remove the RNA protecting reagent, and the pellet was resuspended in 100 µL Tris-EDTA buffer (TE, 1M Tris pH 8, 0.5M EDTA pH 8, dH$_2$O).

For *P. aeruginosa* biofilms, the samples were treated with lysozyme at 4.4 mg/mL (Omega Bio-tek, USA) and incubated at room temperature for 5 min. Then, approximately 25 mg of glass beads (Omega Bio-tek, USA) were added and the tubes were vortexed at maximum speed for 5 min. Cell debris and glass beads were removed by centrifugation at 7224 x *g* for 2 min and the supernatant was transferred to a clean RNase/DNase free microcentrifuge tube. Regarding *S. aureus* biofilms, the samples were treated with lysozyme at 2.5 mg/mL and lysostaphin at 0.1 mg/mL (Sigma-Aldrich) and incubated at 37°C for 30 min.

RNA was then extracted using the GeneJET RNA Purification Kit (Thermo Fisher Scientific, USA) according to the manufacturer's instructions (starting from step 4 onwards). Extracted RNA was immediately purified using the DNA-*free* Kit (Invitrogen by Thermo Fisher Scientific, USA) following the Rigorous DNase treatment protocol provided by the manufacturer. When necessary, purified RNA was treated twice with DNase to remove any residual genomic DNA. RNA concentration (A260/A280 ratio) and purity (A230/A260 ratio) were evaluated using a NanoDrop One spectrophotometer (Thermo Fisher Scientific, USA). RNA integrity of the first samples obtained was also assessed by running the samples in an 1% agarose gel supplemented with 0.5% (*v/v*) commercial bleach, to prevent RNase contamination and consequent RNA digestion, in TAE (Tris-acetate-ethylenediaminetetraacetic acid) 1X buffer (TAE buffer; 40 mM Tris, 40 mM acetic acid, and 1 mM EDTA). Nucleic acids were stained with GreenSafe Premium (NZYTech, Portugal) and agarose gel electrophoresis was performed at 100 V for 60 min using a PowerPac™ HC power supply (Bio-Rad Laboratories, Inc., USA). Purified RNA was stored at -80°C.

7.3. Confirmation of DNA absence in RNA samples by qPCR

The confirm that the previous treatment with DNase was effective in removing all DNA from RNA samples, previously obtained from both *P. aeruginosa* and *S. aureus* biofilms, qPCR reactions were performed, using primers for the housekeeping genes of each species, *rpoS* and 16S rRNA, respectively (Tables 1 and 2). Residual genomic DNA in the RNA samples would conduct to gene amplification and quantification. qPCR was performed using the PerfeCTa SYBR Green FastMix Kit (Quantabio, USA). Each PCR reaction contained 1 µL RNA template, 5 µL SYBR Green FastMix, each primer at

500 mM (Eurofins Genomics, Germany) and nuclease free water to a final volume of 10 µL. A no template control (NTC) was included. Thermal cycling conditions were as follows: an initial activation step of 95°C for 10 min, followed by 40 cycles of 95°C for 15 s and 60°C for 60 s for Taq polymerase amplification. A melt curve analysis was performed at a temperature range of 69°C to 95°C with 0.3°C/s intervals. PCR reactions were carried out in a Q qPCR instrument (Quantabio) and results analyzed through its associated software.

Table 1: Primers used for *P. aeruginosa* ATCC 27853 and Pa3 RT-qPCR analysis.

Gene	Sequence (5' -> 3')	Reference
rpoS	Forward: CTCCCCGGGCAACTCCAAAAG	
	Reverse: CGATCATCCGCTTCCGACCAG	
pqsA	Forward: GTTTCTGGTTCCTACCTGCC	
	Reverse: CAGCAGGATCTGGTTGTCGT	
pqsE	Forward: GGTTGAAGGAGGGATCAGCC	
	Reverse: AGTGGTCGTAGTGCTTGTGG	
pqsR	Forward: GATAGCCTGGCGACGATCAA	
	Reverse: CACTGGTTGAAGCGGGAGAT	(Birmes et
lasI	Forward: CAGAACGACATCCAGACGCT	al., 2019)
	Reverse: TCGATGCCGATCTTCAGGTG	
lasR	Forward: AGATCCTGTTCGGCCTGTTG	
	Reverse: GGGTAGTTGCCGACGATGAA	
rhlI	Forward: CAGTTCGACCATCCGCAAAC	
	Reverse: GACGTCCTTGAGCAGGTAGG	
rhlR	Forward: GTTTGCGTAGCGAGATGCAG	
	Reverse: GGCGTAGTAATCGAAGCCCA	

Table 2: Primers used for *S. aureus* ATCC 29213, SA007 and SA011 RT-qPCR analysis.

Gene	Sequence (5' -> 3')	Reference
16S	Forward: CCATAAAGTTGTTCTCAGTT	
rRNA	Reverse: CATGTCGATCTACGATTACT	
agrA	Forward: ACGTGGCAGTAATTCAGTGTATGTT	
	Reverse: GGCAATGAGTCTGTGAGATTTTGT	
sarA	Forward: GCTGTATTGACATACATCAGCGAAA	
	Reverse: CGTTGTTTGCTTCAGTGATTCGT	(Chen et
RNAIII	Forward: GAATTTGTTCACTGTGTCGATAATCCATTT	al., 2016)
	Reverse: GAAGGAGTGATTTCAATGGCACAAGATAT	
ica	Forward: TCGCACTCTTTATTGATAGTCGCTACGAG	
	Reverse: TGCGACAAGAACTACTGCTGCGTTAAT	
hla	Forward: ATGGCTCTATGAAAGCAGCAGA	
	Reverse: AAGGTGAAAACCCTGAAGA	

8. Evaluation of QS-related genes expression by *P. aeruginosa* and *S. aureus*

8.1. Relative gene expression in *P. aeruginosa* QS-related genes by RT-qPCR

For *P. aeruginosa* ATCC 27853 and Pa3, cDNA synthesis and amplification were performed in a single step using the qScript One-Step SYBR Green RT-qPCR Kit (Quantabio). Each PCR reaction contained 1 µL RNA template at 100 ng/µL, 5 µL One-Step SYBR Green Master Mix, each primer at 200 nM (Eurofins Genomics, Germany) (Table 1), 0.2 µL qScript One-Step Reverse Transcriptase and nuclease free water to a final volume of 10 µL. A no template control (NTC) and a no reverse transcriptase enzyme control (NRT) were included. Thermal cycling conditions were as follows: an initial reverse transcription step at 50°C for 10 min, an activation cycle of 95°C for 60 s, followed by 35 cycles of 95°C for 10 s and 60°C for 30 s. A melt curve analysis was performed at a temperature range of 69°C to 95°C with 0.3°C/s intervals. PCR detection was performed using a Q qPCR instrument (Quantabio). All measurements were carried out in three biological replicates, each in technical duplicates. The PCR detection system software generated the cycle-threshold (Ct) values and relative levels of gene expression were calculated by the ΔΔCt method, using the *rpoS* gene as internal control.

8.2. Relative gene expression of *S. aureus* QS-related genes by RT-qPCR

Regarding *S. aureus* ATCC 29213, SA007 and SA011 gene expression quantification, cDNA synthesis was performed in 1 µg of purified RNA using the qScript cDNA Synthesis Kit (Quantabio) according to the manufacturer's instructions. Then, the amplification step was performed using the PerfeCTa SYBR Green FastMix Kit (Quantabio). The first-strand product was diluted 1:10, and from this dilution, 1/10th was used as template for qPCR amplification. Thus, each PCR reaction contained 1 µL cDNA template at 5 ng/ µL, 5 µL SYBR Green FastMix, each primer at 500 mM (Eurofins Genomics, Germany) (Table 2) and nuclease free water to a final volume of 10 µL. A no template control (NTC) and a control using the purified RNA as template (not subjected to cDNA synthesis) were included. Thermal cycling conditions were as follows: an initial activation step of 95°C for 10 min, followed by 40 cycles of 95°C for 15 s and 60°C for 60 s. A melt curve analysis was performed at a temperature range of 69°C to 95°C with 0.3°C/s intervals. All measurements were carried out in three biological replicates, each in technical duplicates. The PCR detection system software generated the cycle-threshold (Ct) values and relative levels of gene expression were calculated by the ΔΔCt method, using the 16S rRNA gene as internal control.

9. *In vivo* toxicity and infection assays in *Galleria mellonella* larvae

The greater wax moth larvae were obtained from Biosystems (Biosystems Technology, UK). Groups of sixteen larvae in the final instar stage weighing between 180 and 350 mg were used for each experimental condition. Larvae were injected using a 0.5 mL insulin syringe in the last left proleg, into the hemocoel. For the toxicity assay, *G. mellonella* larvae were injected with 10 µL of **B** and **4** diluted in PBS at 25 and 50 mg/kg.

For infection assay, to optimize bacterial concentration, larvae were infected with several different inocula of *S. aureus* ATCC 29213, prepared in PBS as mentioned previously, at concentrations ranging from 1.5×10^8 to 9×10^8 CFU/mL.

Controls included a group of larvae that did not receive any injection and another group of larvae that were injected with 10 µL of PBS. The larvae were then incubated in the dark at 37°C and they were assessed daily for survival for up to 7 days post-injection. Larvae were considered as dead when no movement was displayed in response to stimulation by touch. Experiments were repeated 2 times (16 larvae per group).

10. Assessing the efficacy of **B** and **4** to protect *G. mellonella* against infection by *S. aureus*

Groups of twenty larvae in the final instar stage weighing 180-350 mg were used for each experimental condition. One inoculum of *S. aureus* ATCC 29213 at 4.41 x 10^8 CFU/mL was prepared by adjustment of OD at 600 nm to 0.35. Larvae were infected by injecting 10 µL of the inoculum in the last left proleg and incubated at 37°C for 1 h. After 1 h, infected larvae were treated with 10 µL of **B** at 50 mg/kg or **4** at 25 mg/kg, prepared in PBS, in the last right proleg and incubated in the dark at 37°C. Controls included a group of larvae that did not receive any injection, one group of larvae that were injected with 10 µL of PBS and one group of larvae that were inoculated with *S. aureus* and treated with PBS. The larvae were assessed daily for survival for up to 7 days post-injection. Larvae were considered as dead when no movement was displayed in response to stimulation by touch.

11. Photoactivation of compound **15** and evaluation of its potential bactericidal activity in *S. aureus*

As mentioned above, the compounds from **Group 2** are thought to be activated by light.

To assess the effect of treatment with light in activating these compounds and increasing their antibacterial activity, we have been optimizing the photoactivation protocol. For that, so far, the activity against *S. aureus* ATCC 29213 has been tested and a reference compound, protoporphyrin IX (a molecule known to be activated by light), has been used.

An inoculum of *S. aureus* was prepared in PBS and the OD_{600} was adjusted to 0.1. Protoporphyrin IX, and compounds **15** and **16** were tested so far at concentrations of 200, 100 and 50 µM in PBS. 100 µL of each dilution were transferred to a well of a 96 flat-well microplate to which 100 µL of inoculum was then added. A control well of inoculum and PBS was included. Another 96-well microplate was equally prepared. The plates were incubated at 37°C for 30 minutes. Following incubation, one of the plates was irradiated for 15 minutes using a 25 mW/cm^2 (22.5 J/cm^2) white light, and the remaining plate was kept in the dark. After that, cell viability was evaluated by determining the colony forming units (CFU) of each condition, by plaquing successive dilutions of 10^{-1} to 10^{-6} in agar plates. The plates where then incubated at 37°C for 24 hours. The following day, colonies were counted and CFU/mL were determined.

12. Statistical analysis

The results regarding the inhibition of biofilm formation and quantitative evaluation of violacein formation assays are expressed as mean values ± standard error of the mean. The statistical significance of differences between controls and experimental groups was determined using Student's *t*-test. Probability values (p) of <0.05 were considered statistically significant.

Regarding the relative gene expression quantification assays by RT-qPCR, the PCR detection system software generated the cycle-threshold (Ct) values, defined as the number of cycles required for the fluorescent signal to cross the threshold (when it exceeds background level). Relative levels of gene expression were calculated by the ΔΔCt method, using the *rpoS* or 16S rRNA genes, as internal controls (reference genes) for *P. aeruginosa* or *S. aureus*, respectively, as follows:

$$\Delta Ct \text{ (control)} = Ct \text{ Gene of interest (control)} - Ct \text{ Reference Gene (control)}$$
$$\Delta Ct \text{ (treated)} = Ct \text{ Gene of interest (treated)} - Ct \text{ Reference Gene (treated)}$$
$$\Delta\Delta Ct = \Delta Ct \text{ (treated)} - \Delta Ct \text{ (control)}$$

Results are expressed as ΔΔCt ± confidence interval at 95% confidence. The statistical analysis was performed with R software, considering * p < 0.05 as statistical significance.

Chapter III: Results and Discussion

Results – **Group 1**

1. MIC and MBC values against *P.* aeruginosa, *S. aureus*, *M. luteus*, *S. epidermidis* and *S. pyogenes*

Extracts and compounds of natural/bioinspired origin (**Group 1**) were tested for their antibacterial activity against five bacterial species. As shown in Table 3, overall, compounds and extracts did not affect the bacterial growth (with MIC > or = to 512 µg/mL) of the strains tested. Nevertheless, compounds **0** and **8** and extract C were slightly active against *M. luteus* and compound **0** against *S. epidermidis*. Thus, those showing some activity, showed it against Gram-positive strains and not Gram-negatives. Due to a distinctive structure, Gram-negative bacteria, which possess an outer membrane, are usually more resistant than Gram-positive bacteria that lack that important layer (Breijyeh et al., 2020).

Table 3: Minimum inhibitory concentration (MIC) and minimum bactericidal concentration (MBC) values (µg/mL) of the compounds and extracts from **Group 1** against *Pseudomonas aeruginosa* ATCC 27853, *Staphylococcus aureus* ATCC 29213, *Micrococcus luteus* ATCC 4698, *Staphylococcus epidermidis* ATCC 14990 and *Streptococcus pyogenes* ATCC 19615.

Compound/ Extract	*P. aeruginosa* ATCC 27853 MIC (MBC)	*S. aureus* ATCC 29213 MIC (MBC)	*M. luteus* ATCC 4698 MIC (MBC)	*S. epidermidis* ATCC 14990 MIC (MBC)	*S. pyogenes* ATCC 19615 MIC (MBC)
0	>512 (-)	>512 (-)	128 (>512)	128 (>512)	>512 (-)
1	>512 (-)	>512 (-)	>512 (-)	>512 (-)	>512 (-)
2	>512 (-)	>512 (-)	>512 (-)	>512 (-)	>512 (-)
3	>512 (-)	>512 (-)	>512 (-)	512 (>512)	>512 (-)
4	>512 (-)	>512 (-)	>512 (-)	>512 (-)	>512 (-)
5	>512 (-)	>512 (-)	>512 (-)	>512 (-)	>512 (-)
8	>512 (-)	>512 (-)	64 (>512)	>512 (-)	512 (>512)
10	>512 (-)	>512 (-)	>512 (-)	>512 (-)	>512 (-)
11	>512 (-)	>512 (-)	>512 (-)	>512 (-)	>512 (-)
14	>512 (-)	>512 (-)	>512 (-)	>512 (-)	>512 (-)
A	>512 (-)	>512 (-)	512 (>512)	>512 (-)	>512 (-)
B	>512 (-)	>512 (-)	512 (>512)	>512 (-)	>512 (-)
C	>512 (-)	>512 (-)	256 (>512)	512 (>512)	>512 (-)

2. Inhibition of biofilm formation of *P. aeruginosa* strains

Compounds and extracts from **Group 1** were tested for their ability to prevent biofilm formation, at concentrations of 256, 64 and 16 µg/mL, of *P. aeruginosa* ATCC 27853 and *S. aureus* ATCC 29213 by the crystal violet (CV) assay. The CV binds to biofilm indiscriminately, quantifying live and dead cells, as well as biofilm matrix, which allows the quantification of all biofilm biomass.

The results regarding *P. aeruginosa* biofilm biomass quantification in the presence of the compounds/extracts from **Group 1** are represented in Figure 9. It was observed that compounds **3** (at 64 µg/mL), **4** (at 256 and 64 µg/mL), **11** (at 64 µg/mL) and extract **B** (at 64 and 16 µg/mL) significantly affected the biofilm formation by *P. aeruginosa*.

Compounds **0** (at 16 µg/mL), **1** (at 16 µg/mL), **8** (at 64 µg/mL) and extract **A** (at 64 µg/mL) had a slightly impact in the biofilm formation. On the other hand, compounds **1** and **2** (at 256 µg/mL) formed more biofilm compared with the control, whereas compounds **5**, **10**, **14** and extract **C** did not impact biofilm development at any of the tested concentrations.

Compound 0

Compound 0
Biofilm biomass (OD 595 nm)
Control
256 µg/mL
64 µg/mL
16 µg/mL
*

Compound 1
Biofilm biomass (OD 595 nm)
Control
256 µg/mL
64 µg/mL
16 µg/mL
*
*

Compound 2
Biofilm biomass (OD 595 nm)
Control
256 µg/mL
64 µg/mL
16 µg/mL
*

Compound 3
Biofilm biomass (OD 595 nm)
Control
256 µg/mL
64 µg/mL
16 µg/mL
*

Compound 4
Biofilm biomass (OD 595 nm)
Control
256 µg/mL
64 µg/mL
16 µg/mL
*
*

Compound 5
Biofilm biomass (OD 595 nm)
Control
256 µg/mL
64 µg/mL
16 µg/mL

Compound 8
Biofilm biomass (OD 595 nm)
Control
256 µg/mL
64 µg/mL
16 µg/mL
*

Compound 10
Biofilm biomass (OD 595 nm)
Control
256 µg/mL
64 µg/mL
16 µg/mL

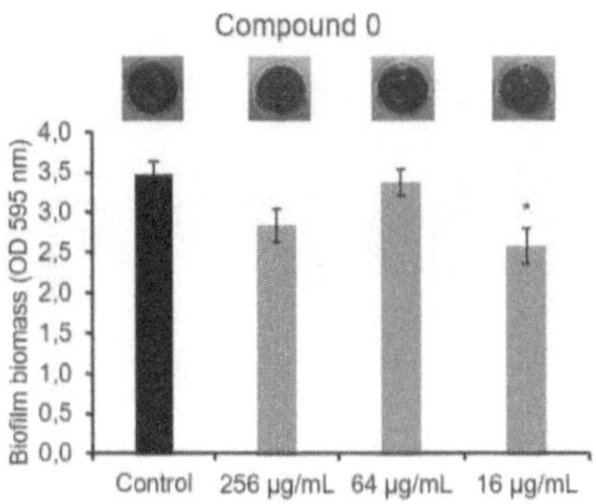

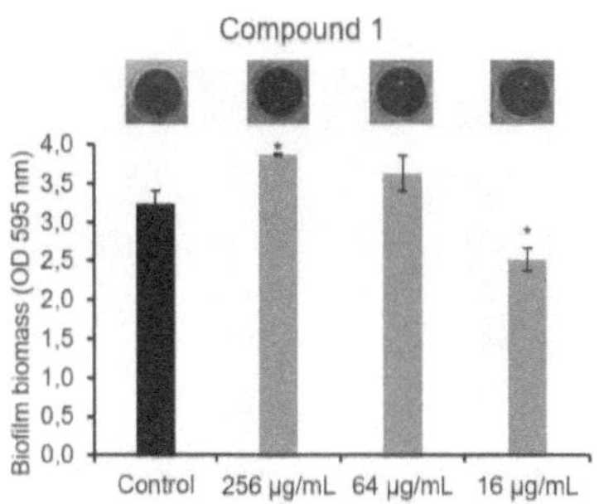

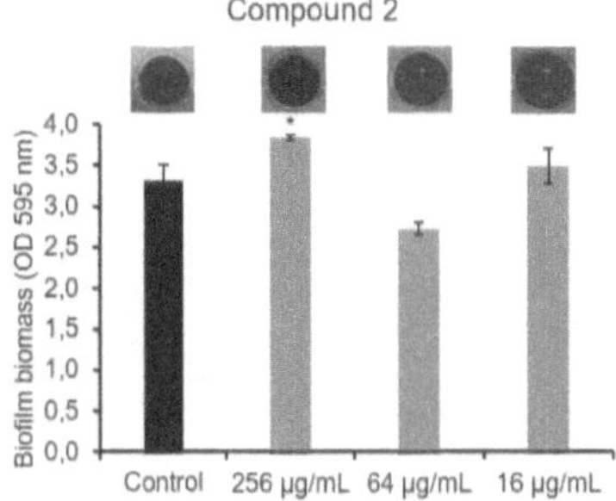

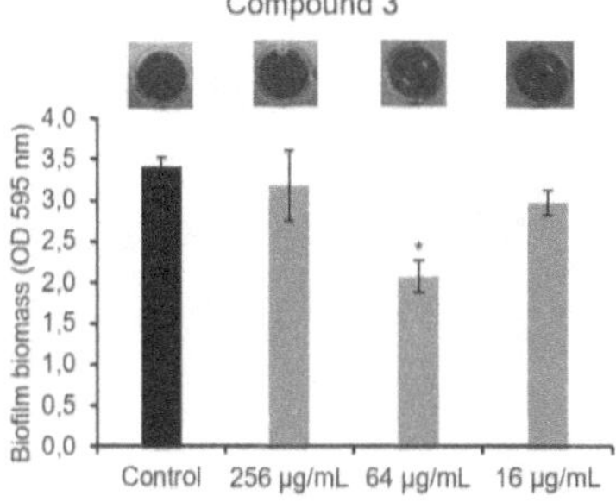

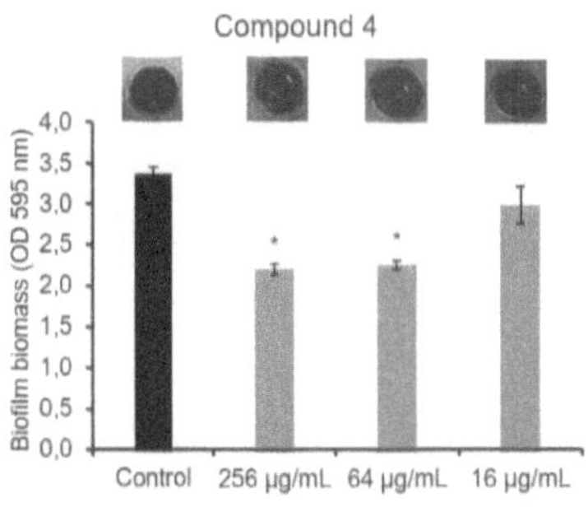

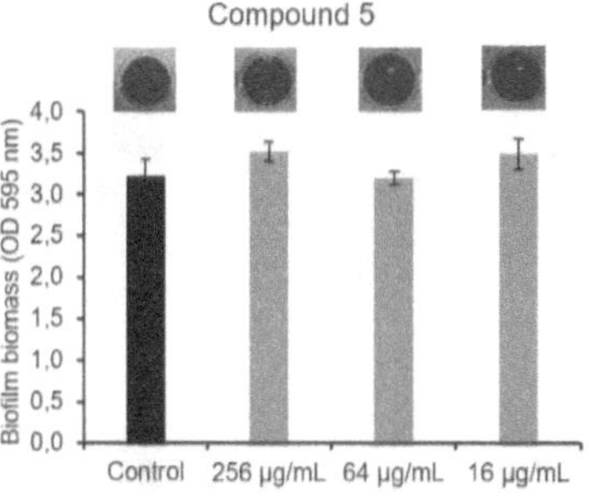

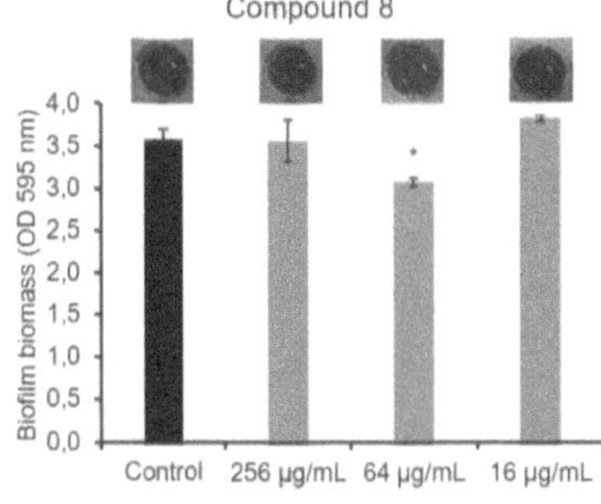

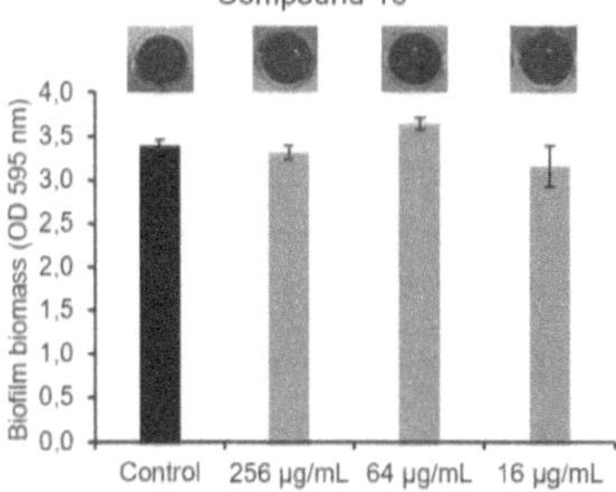

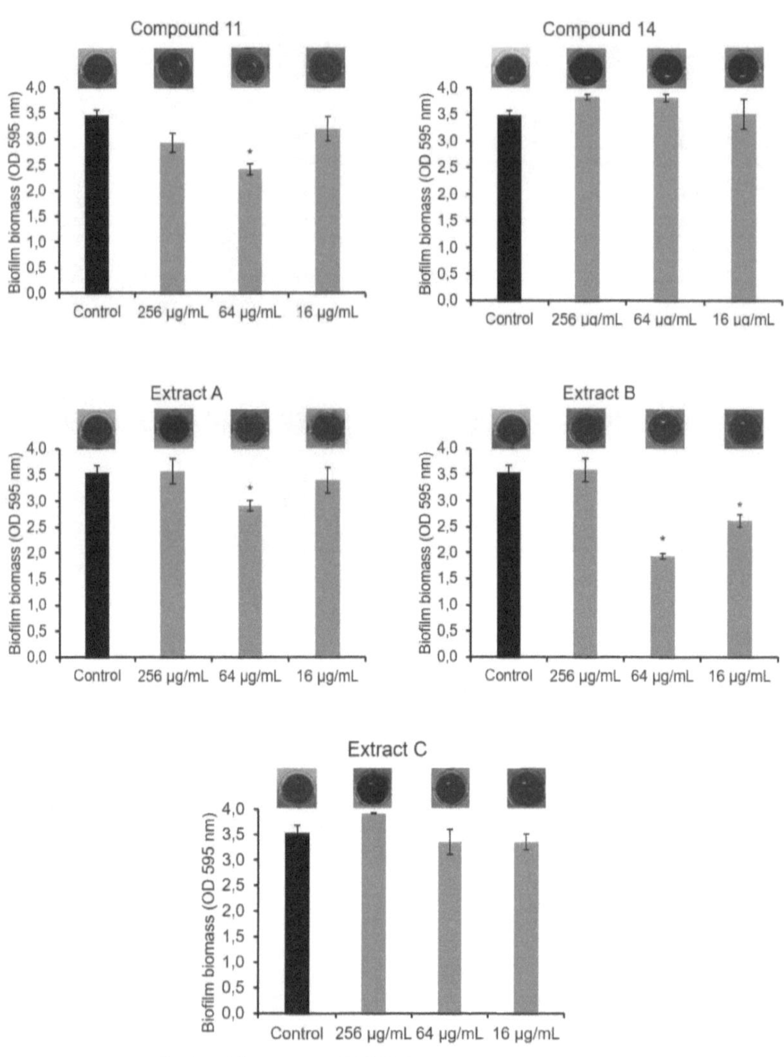

Figure 9: Biomass quantification of *P. aeruginosa* ATCC 27853 biofilms formed in presence of compounds **0** to **14** and extracts **A**, **B** and **C** at 256, 64 and 16 µg/mL, and in absence of any compound or extract (control). Differences between the experimental group and the control were statistically significant when *$p < 0.05$.

The effect of **Group 1** compounds and extracts in *S. aureus* biofilm formation is shown in Figure 10. As observed, compounds **0** (at 256 and 64 µg/mL), **1** (at 64 and 16 µg/mL), **2** (at 256 µg/mL), **3** (at 64 µg/mL), **4** (at 256, 64 and 16 µg/mL), **5** (at 64 and 16 µg/mL), **8** (at 256 and 64 µg/mL), **11** (at 256 µg/mL), **14** (at 256 and 64 µg/mL), and extracts **B** and **C** (at 256 and 64 µg/mL) significantly affected biofilm formation.

On the other hand, compounds **10** (at 256 µg/mL) and **11** (at 16 µg/mL) formed more biofilm compared with the control, highlighting compound **5** (at 256 µg/mL), which showed an accentuated increase in biofilm biomass, whereas extract **A** did not affect biofilm development at any of the tested concentrations. Since the observed inhibition of biofilm formation is not dose-dependent, it can be hypothesized that some of these molecules impair biofilm formation only at optimum concentrations, as previously described in different microorganisms (Gu et al., 2012; Hammond et al., 2014; Sebaa et al., 2017).

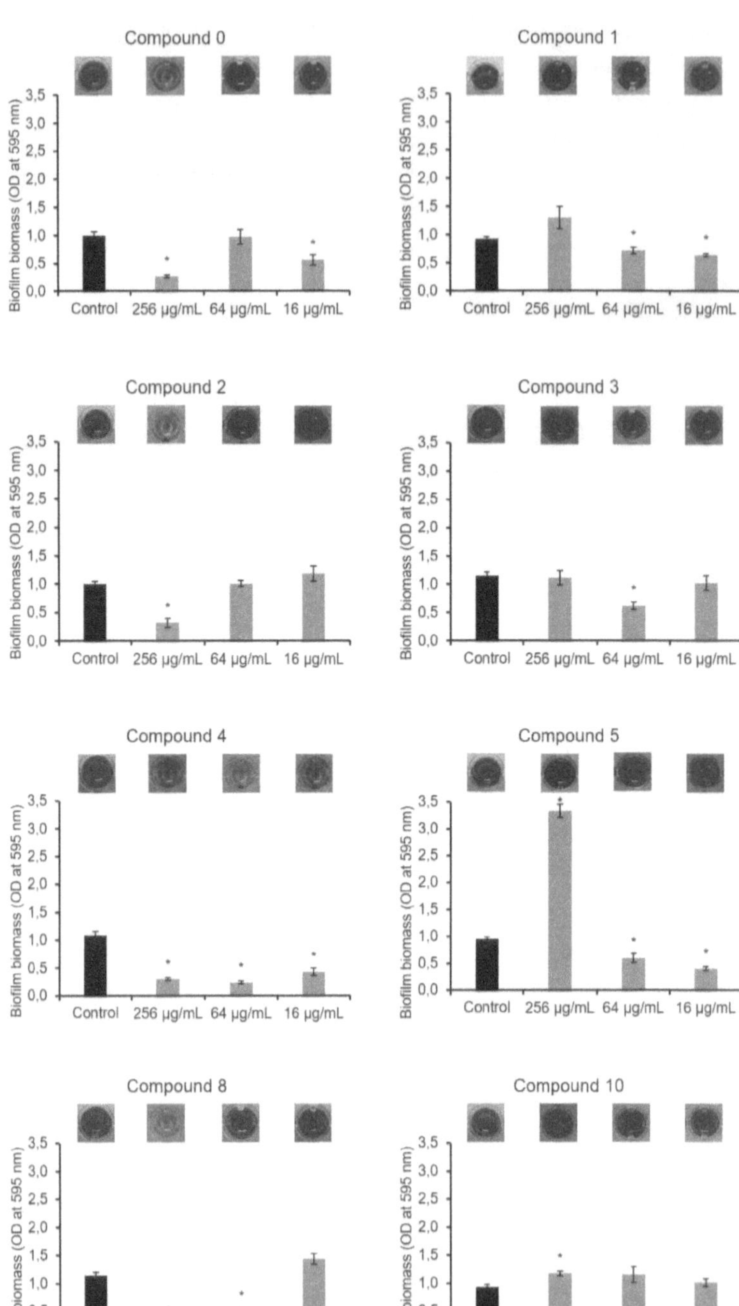

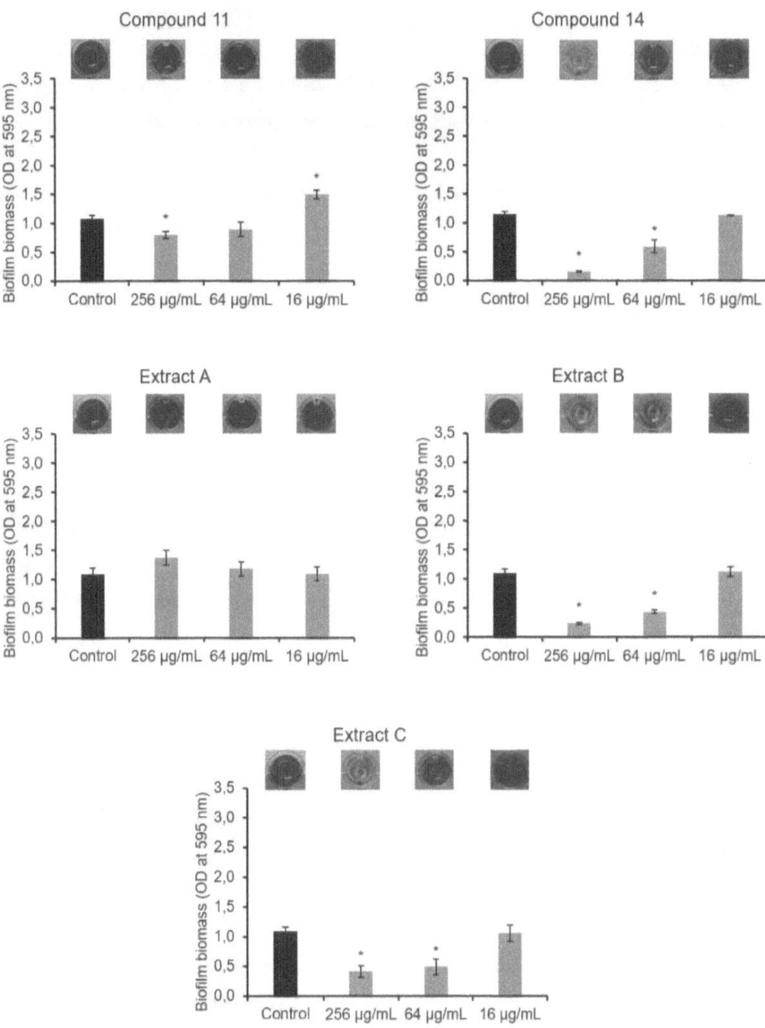

Figure 10: Biomass quantification of *S. aureus* ATCC 29213 biofilms formed in presence of compounds **0** to **14** and extracts **A**, **B** and **C** at 256, 64 and 16 µg/mL, and in absence of any compound or extract (control). Differences between the experimental group and the control were statistically significant when *$p < 0.05$.

We cannot conclude that the increase of biofilm biomass verified in some of the experimental conditions, especially at the higher concentration, is due to promotion of biofilm formation by the compounds. While it may be the case in some instances (**1** and **2** at 256 µg/mL for *P. aeruginosa* and **11** at 256 µg/mL for *S. aureus*), a few compounds seemed to form a precipitate, at higher concentrations, that could not be removed during the biofilm staining protocol, leading to accentuated increases in absorbance values at 595 nm, as observed, for instance, in *S. aureus* biofilms treated with compound **5**.

As we can observe, *P. aeruginosa* ATCC 27853 is a strong biofilm former, while S. aureus ATCC is a moderate biofilm producer (Stepanović et al., 2007).

Taking into account that compound **4** is the main component of extract **A**; compound **11** is the major component of extract **B**; and compound **14** is the main component present in extract **C** and confronting the results obtained for each extract with their main compound, we observed that both in *P. aeruginosa* and *S. aureus*, **C** and **14** showed similar inhibition of biofilm formation, however, **4** had a considerable higher anti-biofilm activity than **A,** and **B** was more effective in inhibiting biofilm formation than its main compound **11**.

These findings may suggest that **4** is more effective in impairing biofilm formation than extract **A**, probably because in the concentration it is present in the extract is not enough to make its activity stand out. On the other hand, the increased anti-biofilm activity of extract **B**, in comparison with its main compound, **11**, indicates that some molecules that compose the extract may be acting in synergy to inhibit biofilm formation in these strains.

Next, based on these results, we decided to select one extract and one compound for further exploring their effects on the biofilm formation of MDR isolates. Due to the promising results in inhibiting the biofilm formation of both *P. aeruginosa* and *S. aureus* ATCC strains, extract **B** and compound **4** were chosen, and tested on the following MDR isolates: PA004, Pa3, SA007 and SA011.

The selected compounds did not affect biofilm formation of both *P. aeruginosa* MDR isolates, which were strong biofilms producers, at any of the tested concentrations (Figure 11). This may suggest that either the compounds' target is altered, inaccessible or absent, or regulated differently in *P. aeruginosa* MDR biofilms. If the target is the QS system, as we anticipate, and knowing that the QS mechanism involves the production, release, and detection of chemical signaling molecules, which permit communication between microbial cells, it is likely that differences between strains may occur in this system regulation upon the presence of these compounds (Lin et al., 2017; Martinez, 2014; Pontes et al., 2018).

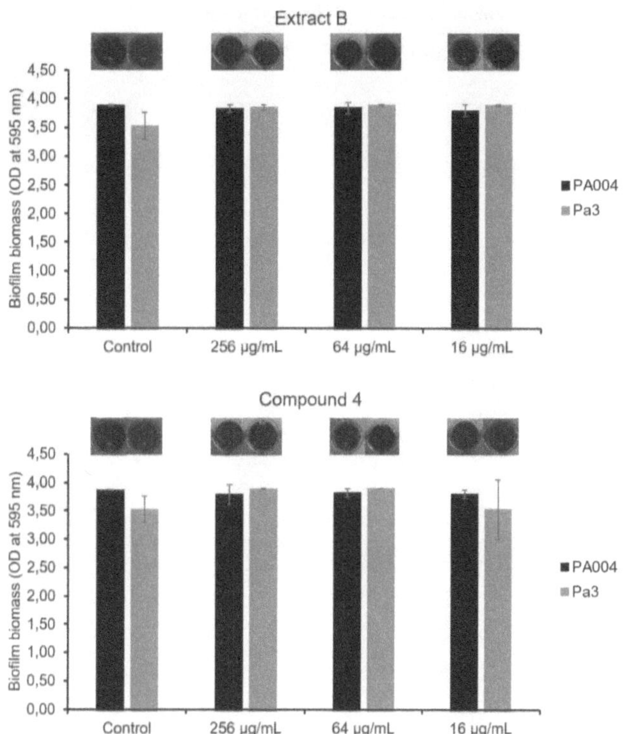

Figure 11: Biomass quantification of PA004 and Pa3 biofilms formed in presence of compound **4** and extract **B** at 256, 64 and 16 µg/mL, and in absence of any compound or extract (control). Differences between the experimental group and the control were statistically significant when *p < 0.05.

In MDR *S. aureus* isolates (moderate biofilm producers), extract **B** significantly decreased biofilm formation at 256 and 64 µg/mL, and in presence of compound **4** significantly less biofilm biomass was quantified is all concentrations (Figure 12).

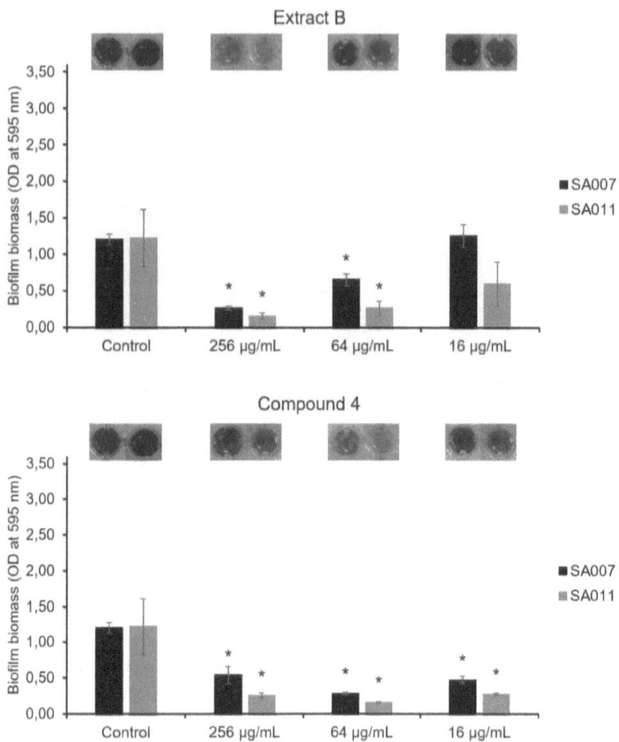

Figure 12: Biomass quantification of SA007 and SA011 biofilms formed in presence of compound **4** and extract **B** at 256, 64 and 16 µg/mL, and in absence of any compound or extract (control). Differences between the experimental group and the control were statistically significant when $*p < 0.05$.

Thus, based on such results and since biofilm formation is QS-regulated (Li et al., 2020), we have raised the question whether these compounds could affect biofilm development by interfering with QS systems. Therefore, extract **B** and compound **4** were then studied for their ability to interfere with the expression of QS-related genes in biofilms of *P. aeruginosa* and *S. aureus*.

3. Effects of **B** and **4** on biofilm formation by microscopic analysis

However, prior to the gene expression assays, and to explore the effects of **B** and **4** at 64 µg/mL on biofilm formation, the live/dead-staining technique coupled with fluorescence microscopy was performed on biofilms of *P. aeruginosa* ATCC 27853, *S. aureus* ATCC 29213, Pa3 and SA011.

Regarding the biofilms of *P. aeruginosa*, we could observe a strong biofilm formation by both strains, either in absence (controls) or presence of **B** and **4** (Figure 13). The biofilm matrix of *P. aeruginosa* ATCC 27853 is composed of three types of exopolysaccharides, alginate, Psl and Pel, which play an important role in the biofilm maturation and development stage (Cao et al., 2017). The *pel* locus refers to pellicle, a biofilm formed at the air-medium interface, which is the type of biofilm formed by *P. aeruginosa* ATCC 27853 (as seen by the naked eye). Those exopolysaccharides matrix components may be responsible for the light scattered seen in the images. Pa3 formed a strong biofilm but with a not so abundant, or probably with a different composition, matrix. As strong biofilms were formed by these two strains, the effects of **B** and **4** could not be properly evaluated, since no significant differences could be pinpointed between those biofilms formed in presence of the compounds or in absence. Even so, biofilms formed in presence of **B** and **4** seemed to be more dispersed, with less cell aggregation. We are aware that an adequate visualization and analysis of these abundant biofilms should have been done in a confocal microscope. However, by the time we were able to do these experiments, we could not have access to a confocal microscope. Nonetheless, we foresee to repeat the experiment and do an observation using confocal laser scanning microscopy (CLSM).

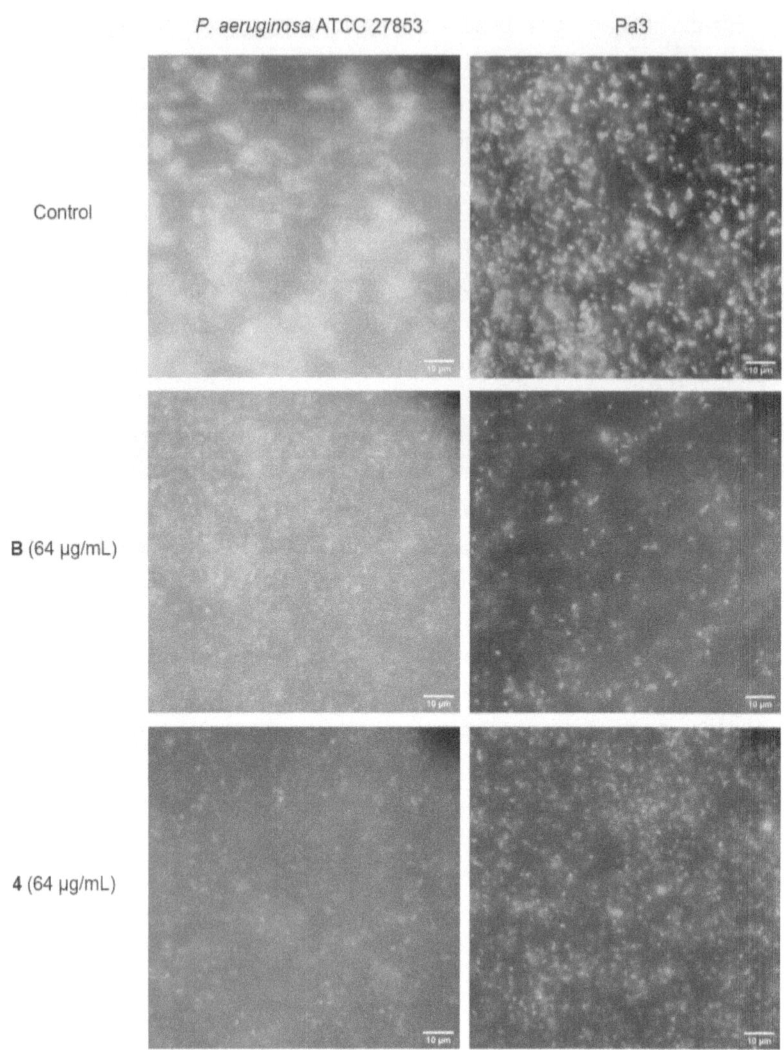

Figure 13: Fluorescence microscopy qualitative evaluation of *P. aeruginosa* ATCC 27853 and Pa3 biofilms formed in absence (control) and presence of **B** and **4** at 64 µg/mL. Representative fluorescent live/dead stain images were obtained after 24 h and depicted here.

Concerning *S. aureus* biofilms, images obtained undoubtedly showed these compounds influenced biofilm formation (Figure 14). In presence of **B** and **4** practically no biofilm was formed, with only a few cells and aggregates adhered to the surface. The results from these observation correlate to those obtained in the crystal violet assay.

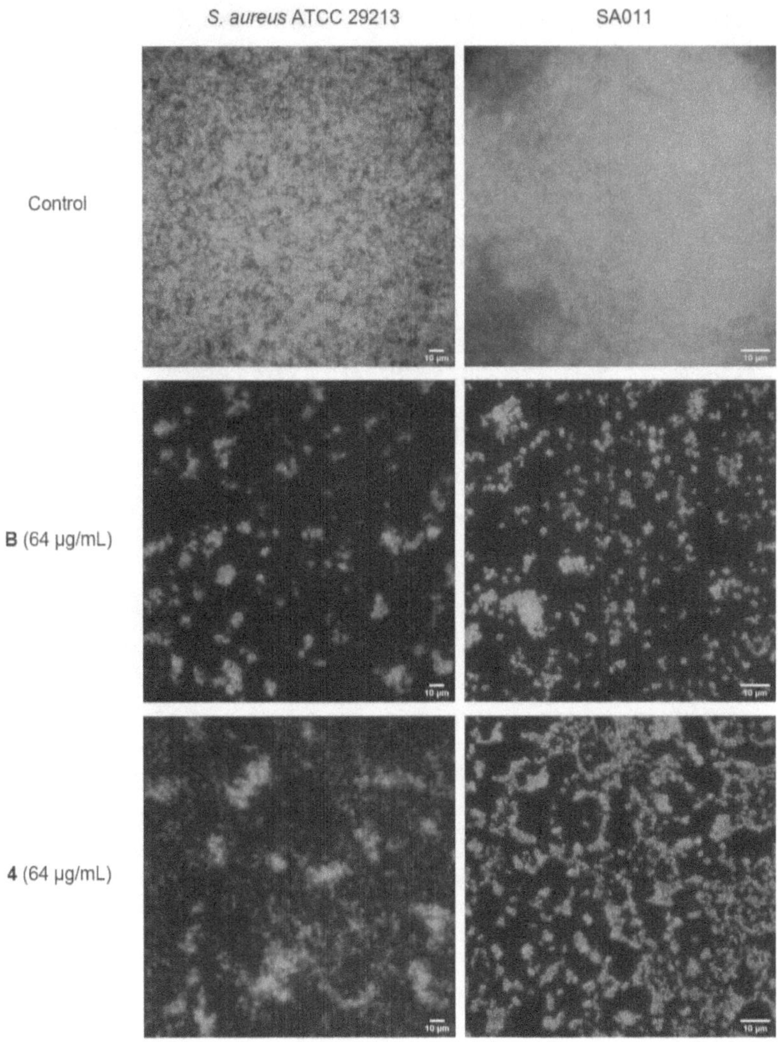

Figure 14: Fluorescence microscopy qualitative evaluation of *S. aureus* ATCC 29213 and SA011 biofilms formed in absence (control) and presence of **B** and **4** at 64 µg/mL. Representative fluorescent live/dead stain images were obtained after 24 h and depicted here.

4. *Quorum sensing* inhibition in *Chromobacterium violaceum* ATCC 12472

Using reporter strains to detect QS inhibition allows high throughput screening of large numbers of drugs (Abraham, 2016).

Anti-QS activity of the ten compounds and three extracts was primarily screened using the reporter strain *C. violaceum* ATCC 12472, which produces a purple pigment, violacein, under the regulation of a QS system. Thus, inhibition of violacein production, observed by a colorless and opaque halo around the discs, indicates interference in the QS.

The compounds and extracts from **Group 1** do not appear to have a strong QS inhibition activity in *C. violaceum*. Nonetheless, **B** and **C**, we could notice colorless colonies near the disc, similar to vanillin (Figure 15). DMSO, which was the solvent of the compounds and extracts, caused a small halo of growth inhibition around the discs.

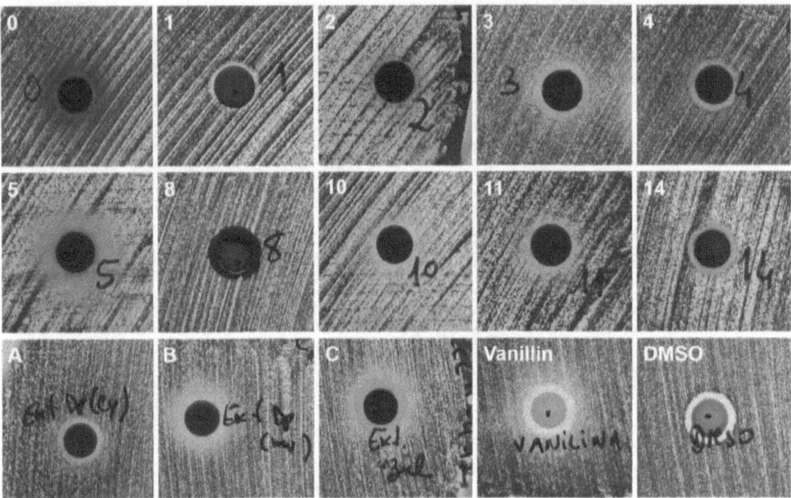

Figure 15: Screening of anti-*quorum sensing* activity of the compounds and extracts on *Chromobacterium violaceum* 12472. Colorless colonies near the disc, resulting from violacein production inhibition, indicate an anti-QS activity. The compounds (**0** to **14**) and extracts (**A**, **B** and **C**) are ordered from left to right. Controls included vanillin (positive control) and DMSO (negative control).

According to the results of biofilm formation inhibition in *P. aeruginosa*, it was expected that **4** would have some anti-QS activity, but that was not verified in this assay. This observation may be explained by the fact that, although they are both Gram-negative bacteria, *P. aeruginosa* and *C. violaceum* have different QS systems, so QS-inhibition occurs in distinct manners. While *P. aeruginosa* harbors the four QS systems described previously in the introduction section, *C. violaceum* QS system consists of the

CviI and CviR components. CviI synthetizes a *N*-decanoyl-L-homoserine lactone (C10HSL) that binds to the receptor, CviR (Kothari et al., 2017). The complex CviR-C10HSL autoinduces *cviI* expression and activates the *vioA* promoter of the *vioABCDE* operon, that encodes the genes for violacein production (Devescovi et al., 2017). It is thought that vanillin acts as a QSI by interacting with the receptor CviR in *C. violaceum* and PqsR in *P. aeruginosa* (Mok et al., 2020). Thus, these compounds may not have the same affinity to CviR as vanillin, but have a higher affinity to the receptors of the *P. aeruginosa* QS systems. Besides, as *P. aeruginosa* harbors more than one QS system, PqsR inhibition alone may not be enough to inhibit QS signaling of this pathogen.

The quantitative determination of violacein production by HPLC (Figure 16 and Supplementary data, Figure S1), showed that compound **4**, that did not seem to influence *C. violaceum* QS in the disc diffusion assay, appears to influence (in a dose dependent manner) violacein production when the pigment was quantified, which corroborates with the results of biofilm formation obtained by the crystal violet assay in *P. aeruginosa*. In fact, the extract and compounds, and their concentrations tested in this assay were selected based on the results obtained regarding the inhibition of biofilm formation by *P. aeruginosa* ATCC 27853. Interestingly, herein compound **3** (at 64 µg/mL) and extract **B** (at both 64 and 256 µg/mL) not only did not inhibit production of violacein but also stimulated its production. Because *C. violaceum* and *P. aeruginosa* harbor distinct QS systems, it is possible that **B** could act as a QSI in *P. aeruginosa* while being an enhancer of the QS pathway that in *C. violaceum* leads to violacein production.

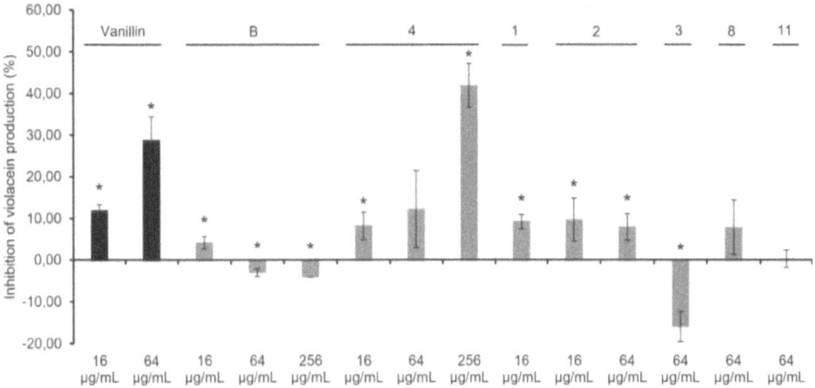

Figure 16: Effect of vanillin, extract **B** and compounds **1**, **2**, **3**, **4**, **8** and **11** on violacein production by *C. violaceum* ATCC 12472. Vanillin, a known QSI, was included as a positive control. Differences between the experimental group and the control (not treated) were statistically significant when *$p < 0.05$.

5. Effects of **B** and **4** in the expression of QS-regulated genes of *P. aeruginosa* and *S. aureus* strains

As **B** and **4** showed promising results in inhibiting biofilm formation by *P. aeruginosa* and *S. aureus* phenotypically, relative gene expression of several QS-related genes was quantified by RT-qPCR for *P. aeruginosa* ATCC 27853, *S. aureus* ATCC 29213, Pa3, SA007 and SA011 biofilms formed in the presence of **B** and **4** at 64 µg/mL.

All protocols were implemented for the first time in the lab, from RNA extraction to genomic DNA degradation and evaluation of RNA purity and integrity, as well as the RT-qPCR reactions. After RNA extraction, a DNase treatment followed, and then the RNA concentration and purity was assessed in a nanodrop (Figure 17) and also through a qPCR reaction to rule out that genomic DNA was in fact not present (Figure 18).

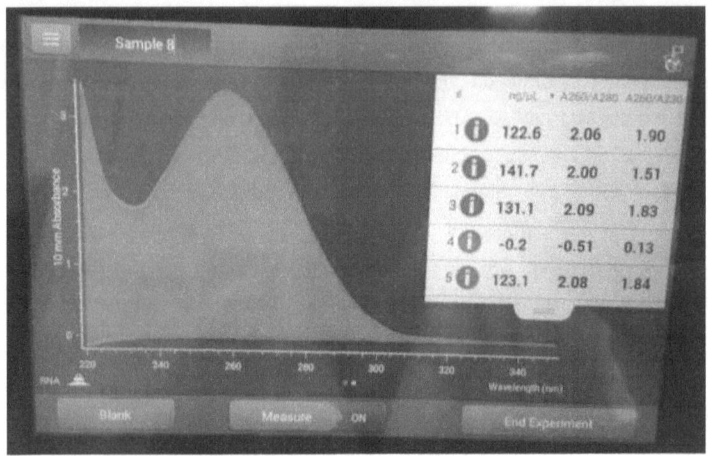

Figure 17: Exemplificative image of the data obtained in the nanodrop measurements.

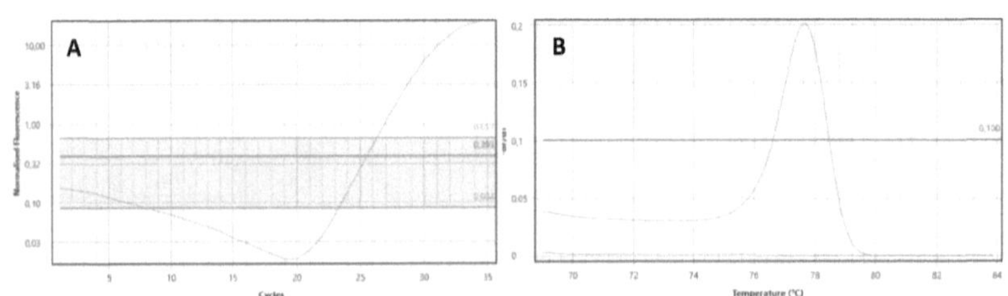

Figure 18: Exemplificative image of the amplification curves (A) and melting curves (B) after qPCR to check if DNA was still present in the RNA samples. The melting curve represented in (B) is above the baseline (red), which indicates that some DNA was still present in the RNA sample.

In cases where some DNA was still present (as the example shown in Figure 18), an additional DNase treatment was performed in the RNA samples and the efficacy of such treatment was further assessed by running another qPCR (Supplementary data, Figure S2).

Initially, in order to be secure about the integrity of the extracted RNA, we have run the extraction product of a few samples in a 1% agarose gel with 0.5% of bleach (Figure 19).

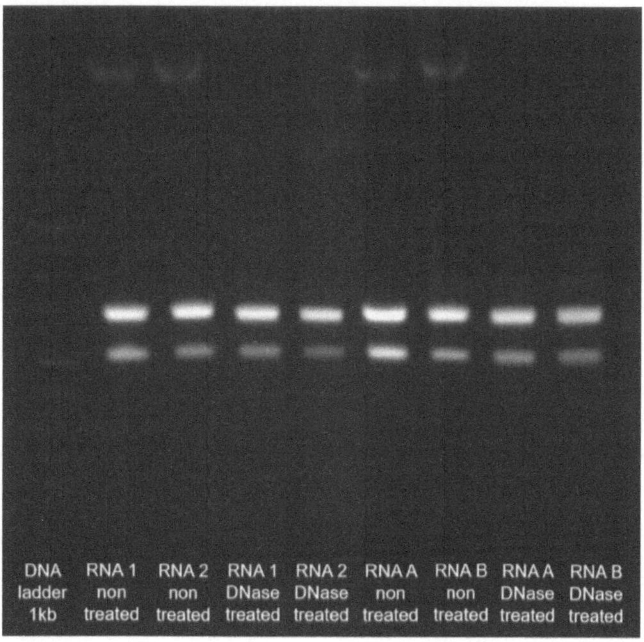

Figure 19: Agarose gel in which samples resulting directly from RNA extraction and from DNase treatment were analyzed. In the samples treated with DNase only the two ribosomal subunits are detected, while in the RNA non-DNase treated is possible to observe the presence of residual DNA.

After all procedures had been optimized, RNA samples of three biological replicates were obtained for each condition (control and treated) and for each strain, and then RT-qPCR was performed in technical replicates for relative quantification of transcription of single genes.

5.1. Effects of **B** and **4** in the expression of QS-regulated genes of *P. aeruginosa*

In *P. aeruginosa* the following genes were assessed: *lasI, lasR, rhlI, rhlR, pqsA, pqsE, pqsR*; and the relative transcript amount was normalized to the *rpoS* internal control gene.

Four main QS systems are present in *P. aeruginosa*, and each one of those systems regulate each other. The LasI/LasR system regulates all other three systems, the RhlI/RhlR and the PqsABCDE/PqsR systems regulating each other, and the AmbBCDE/IqsR system regulating the PqsABCDE/PqsR system (Pérez-Pérez et al., 2017). These systems also regulate the expression of several genes encoding for virulence factors and biofilm formation, etc.

As shown in Figure 20, **B** was shown to significantly downregulate transcription of *lasI* and *rhlI* and upregulate the component of the Pqs system, *pqsE*, in *P. aeruginosa* ATCC 27853. Both LasI/LasR and RhlI/RhlR systems encode for N-acylhomoserine lactones, whose production will be affected upon the presence of **B**. In turn, the RhlI/RhlR system is known to repress/inhibit the PqsABCDE/PqsR system, thus, if the former was affected, the latter system may be activated, explaining the upregulation of *pqsE* gene. The PqsE enzyme is synthase of an autoinducer that activates the QS receptor RhlR (Groleau et al., 2020; Mukherjee et al., 2018). However, herein, the *rhlR* gene was not significantly affected.

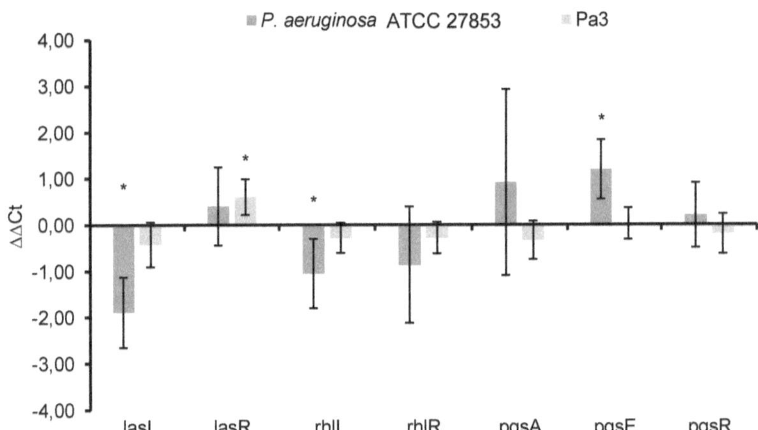

Figure 20: Relative quantification of the QS-related genes *lasI, lasR, rhlI, rhlR, pqsA, pqsE, pqsR* in *P. aeruginosa* ATCC 27853 and Pa3 biofilms formed in the presence of **B** at 64 µg/mL. Results are expressed as ΔΔCt ± confidence interval at 95% confidence. Differences between the experimental group and the control (formed in the absence of extract) were statistically significant when *p < 0.05.

Furthermore, in the Pa3 isolate, treatment with **B** caused upregulation of *lasR* (Figure 20). Because lasR activates the Rhl and Pqs systems (Hemmati et al., 2020), it would be expected that its overexpression would lead to upregulation of *rhlI*, *rhlR*, *pqsR* and *pqsAE*, which was not observed, meaning that an alternative transcription regulator could be responsible for suppressing RhlR and PqsR activation, such as algR or *mexT*, respectively (Kostylev et al., 2019; Okkotsu et al., 2013).

Regarding the effect of **4** in the QS-related gene expression of these strains (Figure 21), **4** proved to downregulate *lasI* and *rhlI* expression, while upregulating *pqsA* and *pqsE* in *P. aeruginosa* ATCC 27853, possibly by the same mechanism observed in the biofilms formed in the presence of **B** (Figure 20).

Whereas in Pa3, **4** downregulated the expression of *rhlI* and *rhlR*, indicating that this compound successfully impaired the Rhl//RhlR system in the Pa3 isolate. As observed in Figure 21, *pqsAER* expression was quite different and even opposite in the two strains. The regulation of this systems is rather complex and the knowledge of is continuously arising and being updated. For instance, LasR-defective mutants have been detected in diverse environments, concretely, it was demonstrated that a lasR mutant isolated from the lungs of a cystic fibrosis patient expressed a *rhl* system that acted independently of the Las system (Chen et al., 2019; Groleau et al., 2020).

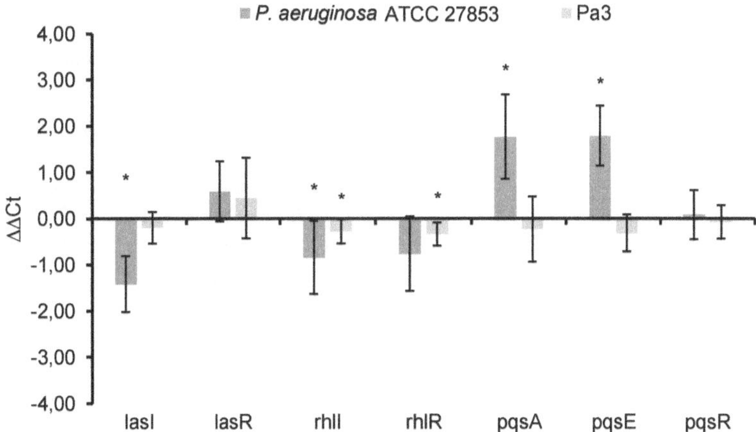

Figure 21: Relative quantification of the QS-related genes *lasI, lasR, rhlI, rhlR, pqsA, pqsE, pqsR* in *P. aeruginosa* ATCC 27853 and Pa3 biofilms formed in the presence of **4** at 64 µg/mL. Results are expressed as ΔΔCt ± confidence interval at 95% confidence. Differences between the experimental group and the control (formed in the absence of extract) were statistically significant when $*p < 0.05$.

5.2. Effects of **B** and **4** in the expression of QS-regulated genes of *S. aureus*

In *S. aureus* the following genes were assessed: *agrA*, *sarA*, *RNAIII*, *ica*, *hla*; and the relative transcript amount was normalized to the 16S rRNA internal control gene.

In *S. aureus*, the *agr quorum sensing* system plays a major role in the regulation of virulence factors production (Butrico & Cassat, 2020). The *agr* operon consists of four genes: *agrB*, *agrD*, *agrC*, and *agrA*. Transcription of the operon is driven by the P2 promoter, which is activated by the response regulator AgrA in an autoregulated fashion. Phosphorylated AgrA also promotes transcription at the P3 promoter, leading to expression of *RNAIII*. RNAIII serves to enhance the expression of genes encoding toxins such as *hla* (α-hemolysin) while reducing the expression of genes encoding surface proteins.

In *S. aureus* ATCC 29213, **B** decreased the transcription of *agrA* (Figure 22), which would be expected to lead to downregulation of downstream genes following *agrA* activation such as *RNAIII* and *hla*, however, that was not observed. Even though the expression of *RNAIII* and *hla* was not significantly affected, *hla* tended to be less expressed, but surprisingly, *RNAIII* tended to be overexpressed.

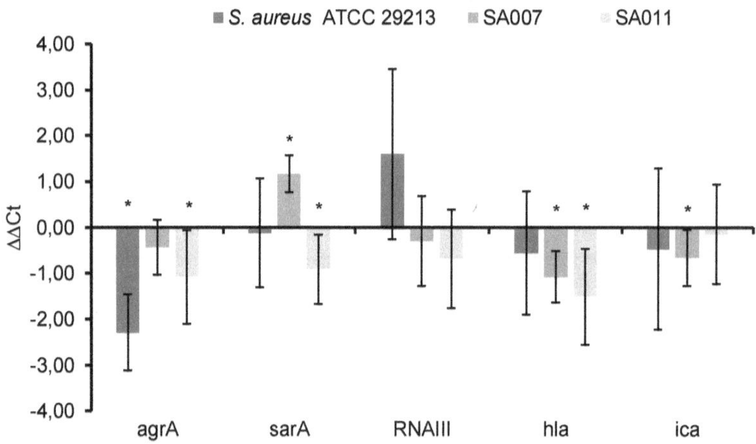

Figure 22: Relative quantification of the QS-related genes *agrA, sarA, RNAIII, ica, hla* in *S. aureus* ATCC 29213, SA007 and SA011 biofilms formed in the presence of **B** at 64 µg/mL. Results are expressed as ΔΔCt ± confidence interval at 95% confidence. Differences between the experimental group and the control (formed in the absence of extract) were statistically significant when *p < 0.05.

In SA007 isolate, treatment with **B** led to upregulation of *sarA* expression and concomitant downregulation of *hla* and *ica*. It would be expected that an increased *sarA* expression would result in increased transcription of *RNAIII*, *hla* and *ica*. The *ica* locus encodes genes required for polysaccharide intercellular adhesion (PIA) production, which is essential for biofilm formation and is under positive regulation by SarA (Omidi et al., 2020). It is possible that a transcription regulator like CodY could be repressing the expression of these genes, despite *sarA* upregulation (Montgomery et al., 2012).

Besides, in SA011, **B** decreased the transcription of *agrA*, *sarA* and *hla*, indicating that this extract could be a potential QSI against this particular MDR isolate, impairing the major QS components.

In *S. aureus* ATCC 29213, **4** activated *sarA* and *RNAIII* transcription and downregulated *hla* and *ica* expression (Figure 23). These results could possibly be explained by repression of *hla* and *ica* by the same mechanism observed in SA007 biofilms formed in the presence of **B**.

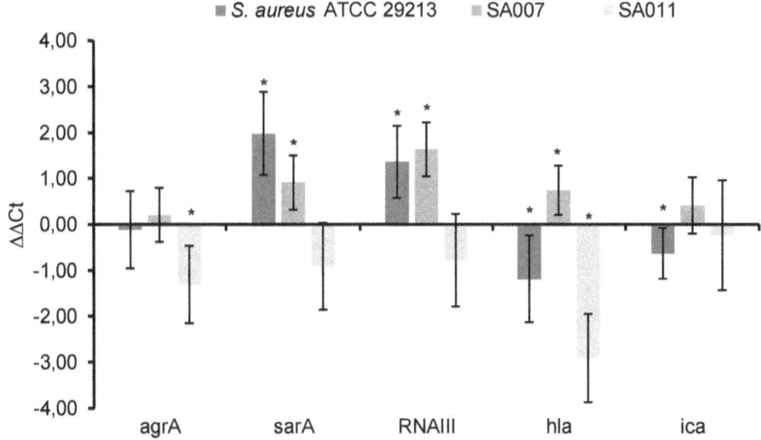

Figure 23: Relative quantification of the QS-related genes *agrA*, *sarA*, *RNAIII*, *ica*, *hla* in *S. aureus* ATCC 29213, SA007 and SA011 biofilms formed in the presence of **4** at 64 µg/mL. Results are expressed as ΔΔCt ± confidence interval at 95% confidence. Differences between the experimental group and the control (formed in the absence of extract) were statistically significant when *$p < 0.05$.

Regarding the MDR isolates gene expression, treatment with this compound resulted in upregulation of sarA, *RNAIII* and *hla* expression in SA007 and decrease of *agrA* and *hla* transcription in SA011. It was proved that AgrA negatively regulates production of proteases that degrade several virulence factors such as coagulases and phenol-soluble modulins (PSMs) (Butrico & Cassat, 2020; Cassat et al., 2013; Kolar et al., 2013). Thus, inhibition of *agrA* in SA011 and consequent protease de-repression might be the reason why biofilm structure is so deeply affected after treatment with both **B** and **4**. However, we observed that SA007 biofilm structure was also affected by **B** and **4**. While **B** might have an impact on biofilm structure by interfering with the *ica* locus expression, which is essential for biofilm formation, the effect of **4** in the SA007 biofilm is still to be elucidated.

Although **B** and **4** contributed to downregulation of some QS-related genes in *P. aeruginosa* and *S. aureus*, there are differences among the various strains within the same species. This suggests that the effect of these compounds might be strain-specific, as specific strain lineages may have different variants of QS components (Feltner et al., 2016b; Lozano et al., 2018; Tan et al., 2018).

6. Toxicity and efficacy assessment of **B** and **4** in *G. mellonella*

Due to its numerous advantages as an *in vivo* model, *G. mellonella* was used to assess the toxicity of **B** and **4**, and to evaluate de ability of these compounds to treat the larvae upon *S. aureus* ATCC 29213 infection.

The toxicity of **B** and **4** in *G. mellonella* was assessed for two concentrations, 25 and 50 mg/kg (Figure 24 and Supplementary data, Figure S3 and Figure S4). As shown in Figure 24, compound **4** proved to have a substantial toxic effect at 50 mg/kg on the larvae, whilst none of the remaining conditions appeared to have significant toxicity in the *G. mellonella* model.

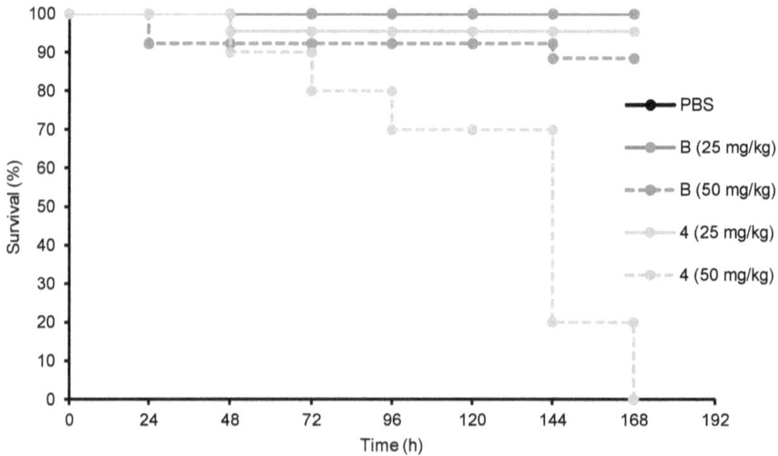

Figure 24: Kaplan-Meier survival-curve of *G. mellonella* larvae injected with **B** and **4** at 50 and 25 mg/kg.

The inoculum was then optimized. The criteria for the adequate inoculum was that it had to kill most of the larvae in 48 h, and all of them in 72 to 96 h. Several inoculum concentrations were tested (Table 4 and Figure 25), and the chosen inoculum was that corresponding to an OD_{600nm} of 0.35 (4.41 x 10^8 CFU/mL), which is turn corresponds to 4.41 x 10^6 CFU/larvae.

Table 4: Optical densities (OD) at 600 nm of the inocula tested and corresponding colony forming units per milliliter (CFU/mL).

OD at 600 nm	Cell counting (CFU/mL)
0.10	1.48 x 10^8
0.20	1.90 x 10^8
0.33	3.20 x 10^8
0.35	4.41 x 10^8
0.40	4.90 x 10^8
0.45	6.20 x 10^8
0.60	8.90 x 10^8

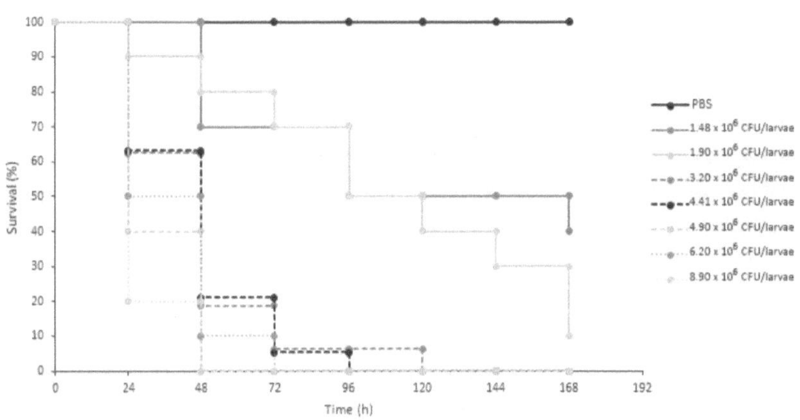

Figure 25: Kaplan-Meier survival-curve of *G. mellonella* larvae injected with several *S. aureus* ATCC 29213 inocula ranging from 1.48 x 10^6 to 8.90 x 10^6 CFU/larvae.

After determining the optimum inoculum, *G. mellonella* larvae were infected with 10 µL of an inoculum of *S. aureus* ATCC 29213 at OD_{600nm} 0.35 (corresponding to 4.41 x 10^6 CFU/larvae), incubated at 37°C for 1 h and then treated with 10 µL of **B** at 50 mg/kg and **4** at 25 mg/kg (Figure 26).

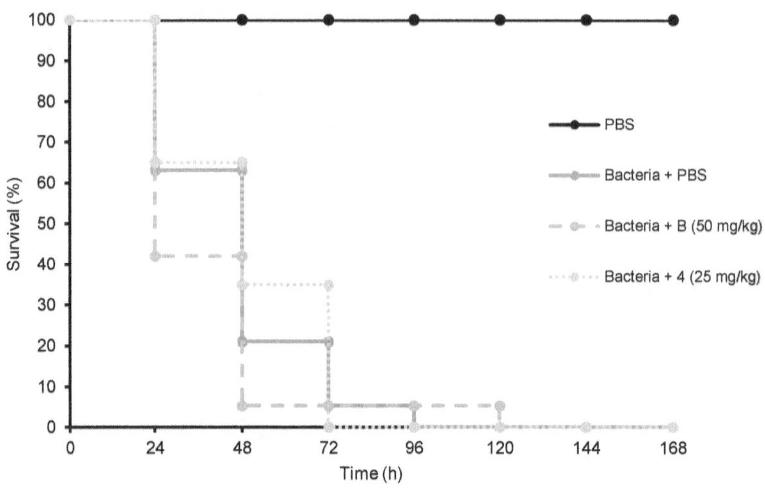

Figure 26: Kaplan-Meier survival-curve of *G. mellonella* larvae infected with an inoculum of *S. aureus* ATCC 29213 corresponding to 4.41×10^6 CFU/larvae for 1 h at 37°C and then treated with **B** at 50 mg/kg and **4** at 25 mg/kg.

As observed, neither **4** nor **B** appeared to have a protective effect on *G. mellonella*'s survival upon infection at the conditions assayed. However, compound **4** seemed to slightly retard larvae's death in the first 72 h. As this experiment was only carried out once, repetition of this experiment is needed to validate the results, and additional infection/treatment experiments with the following adjustments are also necessary: (i) test more concentrations of **B** and **4**, particularly lower concentrations, such as 10 mg/kg, because the compounds activity is not dose-dependent, as verified in the biofilm formation, thus lower concentrations could be more effective against *G. mellonella* infection, and (ii) increase the incubation time to 2 h before treatment, as QS is more prominent at high cell density, 1 h may not be enough for the compounds to exert their anti-QS activity because bacteria may have not reached high cell density in such a short incubation time, which could result in compounds' degradation and metabolization by the larvae before QS has reached its maximum expression.

Results – **Group 2**

7. MIC and MBC values against *P.* aeruginosa, *S. aureus*, *M. luteus*, *S. epidermidis* and *S. pyogenes*

As shown in Table 5, among the compounds from **Group 2**, **15**, **18** and **19** did not show antibacterial activity (MIC > or = 512 µg/mL), except **15** against *S. pyogenes*, causing a MIC of 128 µg/mL. Compounds **16** and **17** showed antibacterial activity, particularly against Gram-positive bacteria, with MIC values ranging from 0.25 to 32 µg/mL, while against the Gram-negative MIC values were of 128 and 256 µg/mL. For **16** and **17**, the MBC values were equal or 4 times higher than the MIC.

Table 5: Minimum inhibitory concentration (MIC) and minimum bactericidal concentration (MBC) values (µg/mL) of the compounds from **Group 2** against *Pseudomonas aeruginosa* ATCC 27853, *Staphylococcus aureus* ATCC 29213, *Micrococcus luteus* ATCC 4698, *Staphylococcus epidermidis* ATCC 14990 and *Streptococcus pyogenes* ATCC 19615.

Compound	*P. aeruginosa* ATCC 27853 MIC (MBC)	*S. aureus* ATCC 29213 MIC (MBC)	*M. luteus* ATCC 4698 MIC (MBC)	*S. epidermidis* ATCC 14990 MIC (MBC)	*S. pyogenes* ATCC 19615 MIC (MBC)
15	>512 (-)	>512 (-)	512 (>512)	>512 (-)	128 (128)
16	128 (>512)	1 (4)	0.25 (1)	1 (1)	8 (16)
17	256 (256)	1 (4)	1 (2)	1 (1)	32 (32)
18	>512 (-)	>512 (-)	>512 (-)	>512 (-)	>512 (-)
19	>512 (-)	>512 (-)	>512 (-)	>512 (-)	512 (>512)

8. Inhibition of biofilm formation of *P. aeruginosa* and *S. aureus*

The compounds from **Group 2** that did not have antibacterial activity (all except **16** and **17**), were tested for their ability to hamper the biofilm formation of *P. aeruginosa* ATCC 27853 and *S. aureus* ATCC 29213, at concentrations of 256, 64 and 16 µg/mL, by the crystal violet (CV) assay.

The effects on *P. aeruginosa* biofilm biomass are shown in Figure 27. It was observed that none of the compounds impaired biofilm formation, except compound **19** that significantly affected biofilm formation at 256 µg/mL.

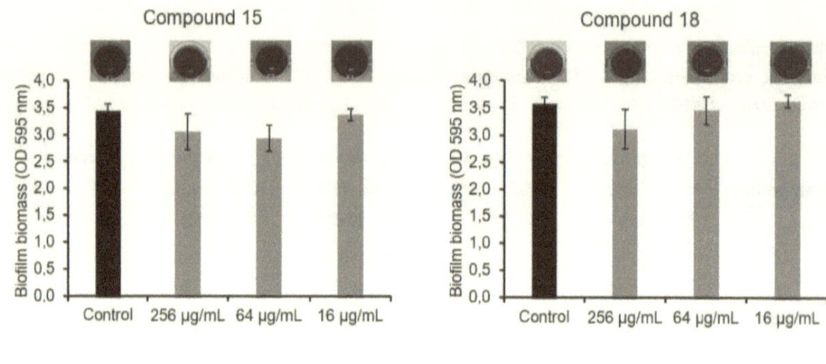

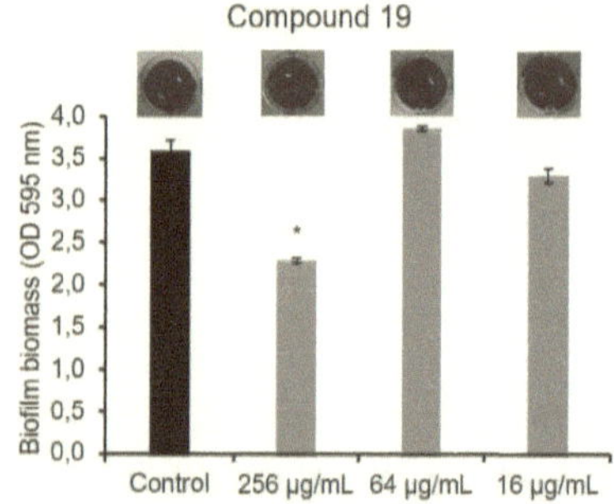

Figure 27: Biomass quantification of *P. aeruginosa* ATCC 27853 biofilms formed in presence of compounds **15**, **18** and **19** at 256, 64 and 16 µg/mL, and in absence of any compound or extract (control). Differences between the experimental group and the control were statistically significant when *$p < 0.05$.

Regarding the effect of compounds of **Group 2** in *S. aureus* biofilm formation (Figure 28), compounds **15** and **19** at 256 µg/mL inhibited it, however, compounds **15** at 64 and 16 µg/mL, **18** at 64 µg/mL and **19** at 16 µg/mL more biofilm was quantified compared with the control.

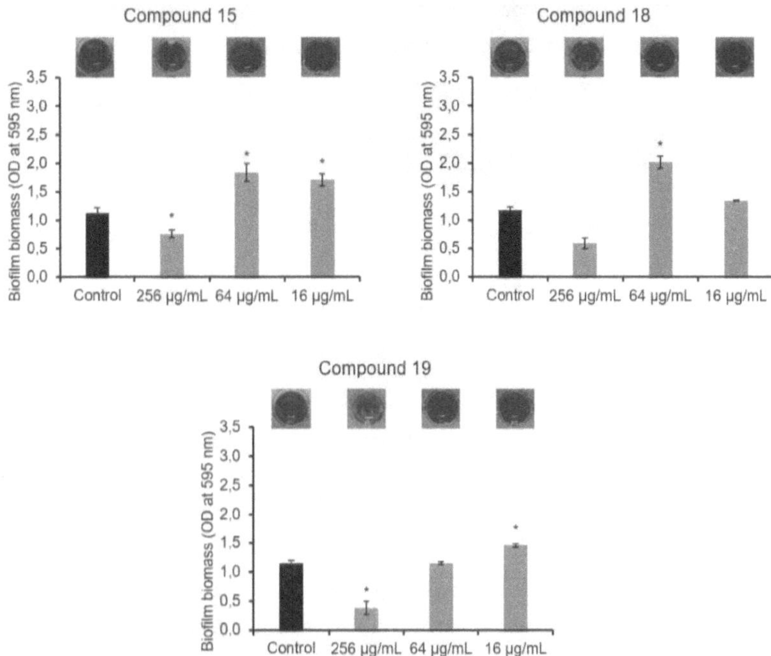

Figure 28: Biomass quantification of *S. aureus* ATCC 27853 biofilms formed in presence of compounds **15**, **18** and **19** at 256, 64 and 16 µg/mL, and in absence of any compound or extract (control). Differences between the experimental group and the control were statistically significant when $*p < 0.05$.

9. *Quorum sensing* inhibition in *Chromobacterium violaceum* ATCC 12472

Concerning the effects of compounds from **Group 2** on QS in *C. violaceum* (Figure 29), it could be observed that **16** and **17**, as expected, caused halos of growth inhibition, indicating that they also affect *C. violaceum* growth. However, the colonies in more close proximity with the compounds were not colorless and, thus, none of the compounds appeared to interfere with QS signaling in this bacterium.

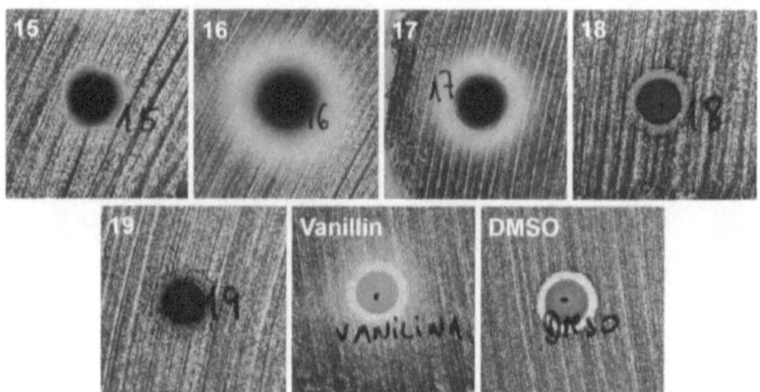

Figure 29: Screening of anti-*quorum sensing* activity of the compounds on *Chromobacterium violaceum* 12472. Colorless colonies near the disc, resulting from violacein production inhibition, indicate an anti-QS activity. The compounds (**15** to **19**) are ordered from left to right. Controls included vanillin (positive control) and DMSO (negative control).

10. Photoactivation of **15**, **16** and Protoporphyrin IX

Since the compounds from this group are believed to be potential photosensitizers, the aim, after assessing their antibacterial activity, was to evaluate if such compounds could be activated by light, in order to develop therapeutic tools against bacterial infections based on antimicrobial photodynamic inactivation (PDI). After light irradiation, the activated photosensitizer can lead to the formation of radicals, which can further interact with oxygen to produce reactive oxygen species. These cytotoxic species can be effective against Gram-positive and Gram-negative bacteria (Ke et al., 2014; Tsai et al., 2011). Thus, we performed an assay to assess the photodynamic inactivation of these compounds on *S. aureus* planktonic cells. Due to the current situation regarding the SARS-CoV-2 pandemic and consequent limitation of laboratory work, this experimental assay was just recently optimized and only compounds **15** and **16** against *S. aureus* ATCC 29213 were tested so far. Incubation and irradiation time, as well as light intensity were previously optimized using Protoporphyrin IX (PPIX), a known photoactivated molecule (Awad, 2014). The results with PPIX in optimized conditions are shown in Figure 30.

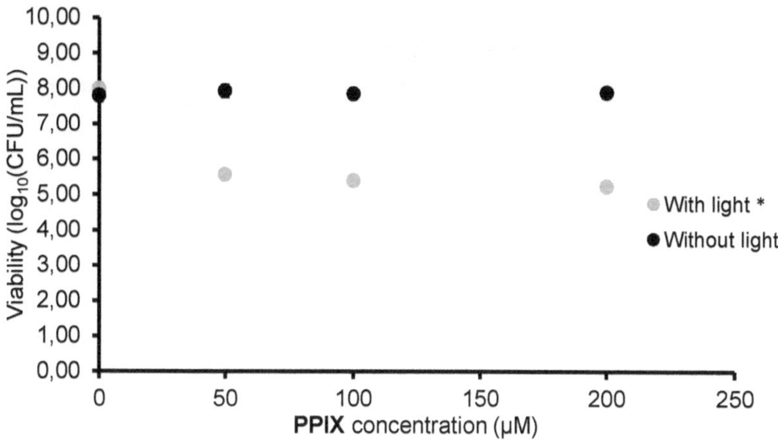

Figure 30: Cell survival fraction of *S. aureus* ATCC 29213 after PDI in the presence of Protoporphyrin IX. Protoporphyrin IX was co-incubated at three concentrations with the bacteria for 30 min and then subjected to illumination at 22.5 J/cm^2 during 15 min. Differences between the experimental group (with light) and the control (without light) were statistically significant when *$p < 0.05$.

As expected, PPIX was activated by light exposure and resulted in a concentration-dependent decrease in bacterial survival. However, the effect of compound **15** on *S. aureus* killing did not seem to be enhanced by light exposure (Figure 31), meaning that it is not activated by light in these conditions or may not be a photosensitizer after all.

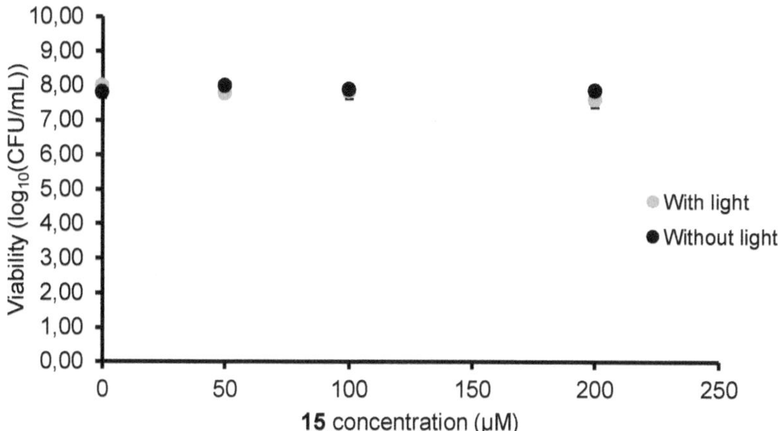

Figure 31: Cell survival fraction of *S. aureus* ATCC 29213 after PDI in the presence of compound **15**. **15** was co-incubated at three concentrations with the bacteria for 30 min and then subjected to illumination at 22.5 J/cm^2 during 15 min. Differences between the experimental group (with light) and the control (without light) were statistically significant when *$p < 0.05$.

Compound **16** previously showed antibacterial activity against *S. aureus*, and therefore a decrease in cell viability can be observed even without light exposure (Figure 32), however, following photoactivation, **16** completely inhibited bacterial growth at all tested concentrations.

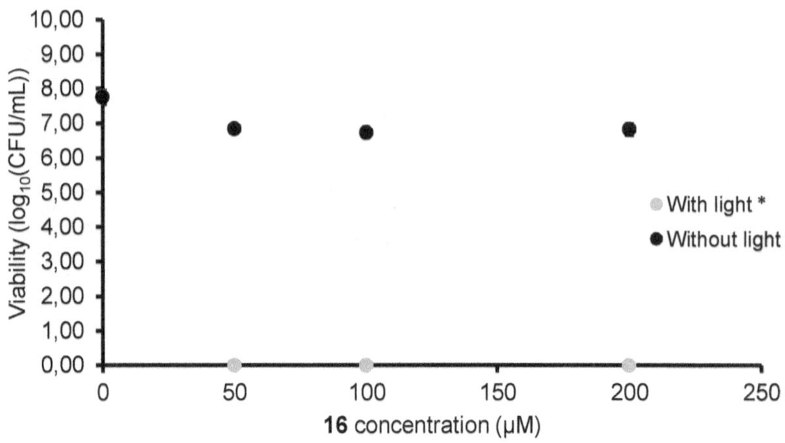

Figure 32: Cell survival fraction of *S. aureus* ATCC 29213 after PDI in the presence of compound **16**. **16** was co-incubated at three concentrations with the bacteria for 30 min and then subjected to illumination at 22.5 J/cm² during 15 min. Differences between the experimental group (with light) and the control (without light) were statistically significant when *$p < 0.05$.

Chapter IV: Conclusions

Most bacteria can become pathogenic due to the production of virulence factors and biofilm formation, and both mechanisms are controlled by a still expanding list of QS systems. Thus, interfering with bacterial QS signaling could represent a promising approach to control bacteria's pathogenesis. Anti-QS agents are able to reduce the expression of virulence genes and were proven to prevent infection in various animal models by enhancing clearance of bacteria.

Here, we explored one compound and one extract of natural origin (whose chemical structure cannot be disclosed due to a patent pending associated to them) that proved to impair biofilm formation and interfere with QS signaling in both *P. aeruginosa* and *S. aureus*. Although their mechanism of action is still to be unraveled, these compounds appear to be promising QSI in both susceptible and MDR strains, and show low toxicity in the *in vivo* larval model *G. mellonella*. Therefore, more studies need to be conducted with several bacterial strains, susceptible and MDR, to assess the potential of these compounds to inhibit QS and prevent infection *in vivo*.

Moreover, in parallel, we were able to increase the bactericidal potential of another set of compounds by photoactivation, which could contribute to the decrease of drug concentration required to treat skin infections.

In sum, knowing the structure of these potential QSI and elucidating their mechanism of action could contribute for the development of stable and effective anti-QS agents that could be applied to the clinical practice and with the potential to not induce the development of resistance. Therefore, these compounds targeting the bacterial QS could revolutionize the way bacterial infections are treated in the future.

However, since QSI have been recently studied and pointed as a good alternative to current antibiotics, their application in the clinic was not seen yet, as most anti-QS agents are still in the preclinical phase. Moreover, an interesting strategy to be pursued would be to combine QSI with antibiotics that could substantially increase the efficacy of both drugs and decrease the cost of medical care.

Chapter V: References

Abisado, R. G., Benomar, S., Klaus, J. R., Dandekar, A. A., & Chandler, J. R. (2018). Bacterial *quorum sensing* and microbial community interactions. In *mBio* (Vol. 9, Issue 3). https://doi.org/10.1128/mBio.02331-17

Abraham, W. R. (2016). Going beyond the control of *quorum-sensing* to combat biofilm infections. *Antibiotics*, *5*(1). https://doi.org/10.3390/antibiotics5010003

Allegretta, G., Maurer, C. K., Eberhard, J., Maura, D., Hartmann, R. W., Rahme, L., & Empting, M. (2017). In-depth profiling of MvfR-regulated small molecules in *Pseudomonas aeruginosa* after *Quorum Sensing* inhibitor treatment. *Frontiers in Microbiology*, *8*(MAY). https://doi.org/10.3389/fmicb.2017.00924

Amato, S. M., Fazen, C. H., Henry, T. C., Mok, W. W. K., Orman, M. A., Sandvik, E. L., Volzing, K. G., & Brynildsen, M. P. (2014). The role of metabolism in bacterial persistence. In *Frontiers in Microbiology* (Vol. 5, Issue MAR). https://doi.org/10.3389/fmicb.2014.00070

Andrea, A., Krogfelt, K. A., & Jenssen, H. (2019). Methods and challenges of using the greater wax moth (*Galleria mellonella*) as a model organism in antimicrobial compound discovery. *Microorganisms*, *7*(3), 1–9. https://doi.org/10.3390/microorganisms7030085

Awad, F. (2014). In vitro Photodynamic Antimicrobial Activity of Protoporphyrin IX in the Presence of Hydrogen Peroxide against *Staphylococcus aureus* and *Pseudomonas aeruginosa*. *British Microbiology Research Journal*, *4*(11). https://doi.org/10.9734/bmrj/2014/10482

Bahari, S., Zeighami, H., Mirshahabi, H., Roudashti, S., & Haghi, F. (2017). Inhibition of *Pseudomonas aeruginosa quorum sensing* by subinhibitory concentrations of curcumin with gentamicin and azithromycin. *Journal of Global Antimicrobial Resistance*, *10*. https://doi.org/10.1016/j.jgar.2017.03.006

Bakar, M. A., McKimm, J., Haque, S. Z., Majumder, M. A. A., & Haque, M. (2018). Chronic tonsillitis and biofilms: A brief overview of treatment modalities. *Journal of Inflammation Research*, *11*, 329–337. https://doi.org/10.2147/JIR.S162486

Balcázar, J. L., Subirats, J., & Borrego, C. M. (2015). The role of biofilms as environmental reservoirs of antibiotic resistance. In *Frontiers in Microbiology* (Vol. 6, Issue OCT). https://doi.org/10.3389/fmicb.2015.01216

Banerjee, G., & Ray, A. K. (2016). The talking language in some major Gram-negative bacteria. In *Archives of Microbiology* (Vol. 198, Issue 6). https://doi.org/10.1007/s00203-016-1220-x

Bäuerle, T., Fischer, A., Speck, T., & Bechinger, C. (2018). Self-organization of active particles by *quorum sensing* rules. *Nature Communications*, *9*(1). https://doi.org/10.1038/s41467-018-05675-7

Bernier, S. P., Lebeaux, D., DeFrancesco, A. S., Valomon, A., Soubigou, G., Coppée, J. Y., Ghigo, J. M., & Beloin, C. (2013). Starvation, together with the SOS Response, Mediates High Biofilm-Specific Tolerance to the Fluoroquinolone Ofloxacin. *PLoS Genetics*, *9*(1). https://doi.org/10.1371/journal.pgen.1003144

Bezar, I. F., Mashruwala, A. A., Boyd, J. M., & Stock, A. M. (2019). Drug-like Fragments Inhibit *agr*-Mediated Virulence Expression in *Staphylococcus aureus*. *Scientific Reports*, *9*(1), 1–14. https://doi.org/10.1038/s41598-019-42853-z

Bijtenhoorn, P., Mayerhofer, H., Müller-Dieckmann, J., Utpatel, C., Schipper, C., Hornung, C., Szesny, M., Grond, S., Thürmer, A., Brzuszkiewicz, E., Daniel, R., Dierking, K., Schulenburg, H., & Streit, W. R. (2011). A novel metagenomic Short-Chain dehydrogenase/reductase attenuates *Pseudomonas aeruginosa* biofilm formation and virulence on *Caenorhabditis elegans*. *PLoS ONE*, *6*(10). https://doi.org/10.1371/journal.pone.0026278

Billings, N., Birjiniuk, A., Samad, T. S., Doyle, P. S., & Ribbeck, K. (2015). Material properties of biofilms - A review of methods for understanding permeability and mechanics. *Reports on Progress in Physics*, *78*(3). https://doi.org/10.1088/0034-4885/78/3/036601

Birmes, F. S., Säring, R., Hauke, M. C., Ritzmann, N. H., Drees, S. L., Daniel, J., Treffon, J., Liebau, E., Kahl, B. C., & Fetzner, S. (2019). Interference with *Pseudomonas aeruginosa quorum sensing* and virulence by the mycobacterial *Pseudomonas* quinolone signal dioxygenase AQDC in combination with the N-Acylhomoserine lactone lactonase QSDA. *Infection and Immunity*, *87*(10). https://doi.org/10.1128/IAI.00278-19

Boles, B. R., & Horswill, A. R. (2008). *agr*-mediated dispersal of *Staphylococcus aureus* biofilms. *PLoS Pathogens*, *4*(4). https://doi.org/10.1371/journal.ppat.1000052

Breijyeh, Z., Jubeh, B., & Karaman, R. (2020). Resistance of gram-negative bacteria to current antibacterial agents and approaches to resolve it. *Molecules*, *25*(6). https://doi.org/10.3390/molecules25061340

Butrico, C. E., & Cassat, J. E. (2020). *Quorum sensing* and toxin production in *Staphylococcus aureus* osteomyelitis: Pathogenesis and paradox. *Toxins*, *12*(8), 1–22. https://doi.org/10.3390/toxins12080516

Cao, H., Lai, Y., Bougouffa, S., Xu, Z., & Yan, A. (2017). Comparative genome and transcriptome analysis reveals distinctive surface characteristics and unique physiological potentials of *Pseudomonas aeruginosa* ATCC 27853. *BMC Genomics*, *18*(1). https://doi.org/10.1186/s12864-017-3842-z

Capilato, J. N., Philippi, S. v., Reardon, T., McConnell, A., Oliver, D. C., Warren, A., Adams, J. S., Wu, C., & Perez, L. J. (2017). Development of a novel series of non-natural triaryl agonists and antagonists of the *Pseudomonas aeruginosa* LasR *quorum sensing* receptor. *Bioorganic and Medicinal Chemistry*, *25*(1). https://doi.org/10.1016/j.bmc.2016.10.021

Cassat, J. E., Hammer, N. D., Campbell, J. P., Benson, M. A., Perrien, D. S., Mrak, L. N., Smeltzer, M. S., Torres, V. J., & Skaar, E. P. (2013). A secreted bacterial protease tailors the *Staphylococcus aureus* virulence repertoire to modulate bone remodeling during osteomyelitis. *Cell Host and Microbe*, *13*(6). https://doi.org/10.1016/j.chom.2013.05.003

Chabelskaya, S., Bordeau, V., & Felden, B. (2014). Dual RNA regulatory control of a *Staphylococcus aureus* virulence factor. *Nucleic Acids Research*, *42*(8). https://doi.org/10.1093/nar/gku119

Chen, R., Déziel, E., Groleau, M. C., Schaefer, A. L., & Greenberg, E. P. (2019). Social cheating in a *Pseudomonas aeruginosa quorum-sensing* variant. In *Proceedings of the National Academy of Sciences of the United States of America* (Vol. 116, Issue 14). https://doi.org/10.1073/pnas.1819801116

Chen, Y., Liu, T., Wang, K., Hou, C., Cai, S., Huang, Y., Du, Z., Huang, H., Kong, J., & Chen, Y. (2016). Baicalein inhibits *Staphylococcus aureus* biofilm formation and the quorum sensing system in vitro. *PLoS ONE*, *11*(4), 1–18. https://doi.org/10.1371/journal.pone.0153468

Chow, J. Y., Yang, Y., Tay, S. B., Chua, K. L., & Yew, W. S. (2014). Disruption of biofilm formation by the human pathogen *Acinetobacter baumannii* using engineered quorum-quenching lactonases. *Antimicrobial Agents and Chemotherapy*, *58*(3). https://doi.org/10.1128/AAC.02410-13

Christensen, L. D., van Gennip, M., Jakobsen, T. H., Alhede, M., Hougen, H. P., Høiby, N., Bjarnsholt, T., & Givskov, M. (2012). Synergistic antibacterial efficacy of early combination treatment with tobramycin and *quorum-sensing* inhibitors against *Pseudomonas aeruginosa* in an intraperitoneal foreign-body infection mouse model. *Journal of Antimicrobial Chemotherapy*, *67*(5). https://doi.org/10.1093/jac/dks002

Cockerill, F. R., Wiker, M. A., Alder, J., Dudley, M. N., Eliopoulos, G. M., Ferraro, M. J., Hardy, D. J., Hecht, D. W., Hindler, J. A., Patel, J. B., Powell, M., Swenson, J. M., Thomson, R. B., Traczewski, M. M., Turnidge, J. D., Weinstein, M. P.(2012). Methods for Dilution Antimicrobial Susceptibility Tests for Bacteria That Grow Aerobically; Approved Standard — Ninth Edition. In *Methods for Dilution Antimicrobial Susceptibility Tests for Bacteria That Grow Aerobically; Approved Standar- Ninth Edition* (Vol. 32, Issue 2).

Conlon, B. P., Rowe, S. E., & Lewis, K. (2015). Persister cells in biofilm associated infections. *Advances in Experimental Medicine and Biology*, *831*. https://doi.org/10.1007/978-3-319-09782-4_1

Cools, F., Torfs, E., Aizawa, J., Vanhoutte, B., Maes, L., Caljon, G., Delputte, P., Cappoen, D., & Cos, P. (2019). Optimization and characterization of a *Galleria mellonella* larval infection model for virulence studies and the evaluation of therapeutics against *Streptococcus pneumoniae*. *Frontiers in Microbiology*, *10*(FEB), 1–11. https://doi.org/10.3389/fmicb.2019.00311

Copitch, J. L., Whitehead, R. N., & Webber, M. A. (2010). Prevalence of decreased susceptibility to triclosan in *Salmonella enterica* isolates from animals and humans and association with multiple drug resistance. *International Journal of Antimicrobial Agents*, *36*(3). https://doi.org/10.1016/j.ijantimicag.2010.04.012

Costerton, J. W., Cheng, K. J., Geesey, G. G., Ladd, T. I., Nickel, J. C., Dasgupta, M., & Marrie, T. J. (1987). Bacterial biofilms in nature and disease. In *Annual review of microbiology* (Vol. 41). https://doi.org/10.1146/annurev.mi.41.100187.002251

Daddi Oubekka, S., Briandet, R., Fontaine-Aupart, M. P., & Steenkeste, K. (2012). Correlative time-resolved fluorescence microscopy to assess antibiotic diffusion-reaction in biofilms. *Antimicrobial Agents and Chemotherapy*, *56*(6). https://doi.org/10.1128/AAC.00216-12

Dastgheyb, S. S., Villaruz, A. E., Le, K. Y., Tan, V. Y., Duong, A. C., Chatterjee, S. S., Cheung, G. Y. C., Joo, H. S., Hickok, N. J., & Otto, M. (2015). Role of phenol-soluble modulins in formation of *Staphylococcus aureus* biofilms in synovial fluid. *Infection and Immunity*, *83*(7). https://doi.org/10.1128/IAI.00394-15

de Vos, W. M. (2015). Microbial biofilms and the human intestinal microbiome. In *npj Biofilms and Microbiomes* (Vol. 1). https://doi.org/10.1038/npjbiofilms.2015.5

Defoirdt, T. (2018). *Quorum-Sensing* Systems as Targets for Antivirulence Therapy. *Trends in Microbiology*, *26*(4), 313–328. https://doi.org/10.1016/j.tim.2017.10.005

Defoirdt, T., Darshanee Ruwandeepika, H. A., Karunasagar, I., Boon, N., & Bossier, P. (2010). *Quorum sensing* negatively regulates chitinase in *Vibrio harveyi*. *Environmental Microbiology Reports*, *2*(1). https://doi.org/10.1111/j.1758-2229.2009.00043.x

Devescovi, G., Kojic, M., Covaceuszach, S., Cámara, M., Williams, P., Bertani, I., Subramoni, S., & Venturi, V. (2017). Negative regulation of violacein biosynthesis in *Chromobacterium violaceum*. *Frontiers in Microbiology*, *8*(MAR), 1–11. https://doi.org/10.3389/fmicb.2017.00349

Dodds, D. R. (2017). Antibiotic resistance: A current epilogue. *Biochemical Pharmacology*, *134*, 139–146. https://doi.org/10.1016/j.bcp.2016.12.005

Dusane, D. H., Zinjarde, S. S., Venugopalan, V. P., McLean, R. J. C., Weber, M. M., & Rahman, P. K. S. M. (2010). *Quorum sensing*: Implications on rhamnolipid biosurfactant production. *Biotechnology and Genetic Engineering Reviews*, *27*(1). https://doi.org/10.1080/02648725.2010.10648149

El-Mowafy, S. A., Shaaban, M. I., & Abd El Galil, K. H. (2014). Sodium ascorbate as a *quorum sensing* inhibitor of *Pseudomonas aeruginosa*. *Journal of Applied Microbiology*, *117*(5). https://doi.org/10.1111/jam.12631

European Centre for Disease Prevention and Control. (2018). Surveillance of antimicrobial resistance in Europe Annual report of the European Antimicrobial Resistance Surveillance Network (EARS-Net) 2017. In *ECDC: Surveillance Report*. https://ecdc.europa.eu/sites/portal/files/documents/EARS-Net-report-2017-update-jan-2019.pdf%0Ahttps://ecdc.europa.eu/en/publications-data/antimicrobial-resistance-surveillance-europe-2016

Fan, X., Liang, M., Wang, L., Chen, R., Li, H., & Liu, X. (2017). Aii810, a novel cold-adapted N-acylhomoserine lactonase discovered in a metagenome, can strongly attenuate *Pseudomonas aeruginosa* virulence factors and biofilm formation. *Frontiers in Microbiology*, *8*(OCT). https://doi.org/10.3389/fmicb.2017.01950

Fedhila, S., Buisson, C., Dussurget, O., Serror, P., Glomski, I. J., Liehl, P., Lereclus, D., & Nielsen-LeRoux, C. (2010). Comparative analysis of the virulence of invertebrate and mammalian pathogenic bacteria in the oral insect infection model *Galleria mellonella*. *Journal of Invertebrate Pathology*, *103*(1), 24–29. https://doi.org/10.1016/j.jip.2009.09.005

Feltner, J. B., Wolter, D. J., Pope, C. E., Groleau, M. C., Smalley, N. E., Greenberg, E. P., Mayer-Hamblett, N., Burns, J., Déziel, E., Hoffman, L. R., & Dandekar, A. A. (2016). LasR variant cystic fibrosis isolates reveal an adaptable *quorum-sensing* hierarchy in *Pseudomonas aeruginosa*. *MBio*, *7*(5), 1–9. https://doi.org/10.1128/mBio.01513-16

Flemming, H. C., & Wingender, J. (2010). The biofilm matrix. In *Nature Reviews Microbiology* (Vol. 8, Issue 9). https://doi.org/10.1038/nrmicro2415

Flemming, H. C., Wingender, J., Szewzyk, U., Steinberg, P., Rice, S. A., & Kjelleberg, S. (2016). Biofilms: An emergent form of bacterial life. *Nature Reviews Microbiology*, *14*(9), 563–575. https://doi.org/10.1038/nrmicro.2016.94

Fong, J., Yuan, M., Jakobsen, T. H., Mortensen, K. T., Delos Santos, M. M. S., Chua, S. L., Yang, L., Tan, C. H., Nielsen, T. E., & Givskov, M. (2017). Disulfide Bond-Containing Ajoene Analogues as Novel *Quorum Sensing* Inhibitors of *Pseudomonas aeruginosa*. *Journal of Medicinal Chemistry*, *60*(1). https://doi.org/10.1021/acs.jmedchem.6b01025

France, M. T., Cornea, A., Kehlet-Delgado, H., & Forney, L. J. (2019). Spatial structure facilitates the accumulation and persistence of antibiotic-resistant mutants in biofilms. *Evolutionary Applications*, *12*(3). https://doi.org/10.1111/eva.12728

Freires, I. A., Sardi, J. de C. O., de Castro, R. D., & Rosalen, P. L. (2017). Alternative Animal and Non-Animal Models for Drug Discovery and Development: Bonus or Burden? *Pharmaceutical Research*, *34*(4). https://doi.org/10.1007/s11095-016-2069-z

Friman, V. P., Diggle, S. P., & Buckling, A. (2013). Protist predation can favour cooperation within bacterial species. *Biology Letters*, *9*(5). https://doi.org/10.1098/rsbl.2013.0548

Furiga, A., Lajoie, B., Hage, S. el, Baziard, G., & Roques, C. (2016). Impairment of *Pseudomonas aeruginosa* biofilm resistance to antibiotics by combining the drugs with a new *quorum-sensing* inhibitor. *Antimicrobial Agents and Chemotherapy*, *60*(3). https://doi.org/10.1128/AAC.02533-15

García-Contreras, R., Nuñez-López, L., Jasso-Chávez, R., Kwan, B. W., Belmont, J. A., Rangel-Vega, A., Maeda, T., & Wood, T. K. (2015). *Quorum sensing* enhancement of the stress response promotes resistance to quorum quenching and prevents social cheating. *ISME Journal*, *9*(1). https://doi.org/10.1038/ismej.2014.98

Glavis-Bloom, J., Muhammed, M., & Mylonakis, E. (2012). Of model hosts and man: Using *Caenorhabditis elegans*, *Drosophila melanogaster* and *Galleria mellonella* as model hosts for infectious disease research. *Advances in Experimental Medicine and Biology, 710*. https://doi.org/10.1007/978-1-4419-5638-5_2

Grandclément, C., Tannières, M., Moréra, S., Dessaux, Y., & Faure, D. (2015). Quorum quenching: Role in nature and applied developments. *FEMS Microbiology Reviews, 40*(1), 86–116. https://doi.org/10.1093/femsre/fuv038

Groleau, M.-C., de Oliveira Pereira, T., Dekimpe, V., & Déziel, E. (2020). PqsE Is Essential for RhlR-Dependent Quorum Sensing Regulation in *Pseudomonas aeruginosa. MSystems, 5*(3). https://doi.org/10.1128/msystems.00194-20

Gu, H., Fan, D., Gao, J., Zou, W., Peng, Z., Zhao, Z., Ling, J., & Legeros, R. Z. (2012). Effect of ZnCl 2 on plaque growth and biofilm vitality. *Archives of Oral Biology, 57*(4). https://doi.org/10.1016/j.archoralbio.2011.10.001

Guendouze, A., Plener, L., Bzdrenga, J., Jacquet, P., Rémy, B., Elias, M., Lavigne, J. P., Daudé, D., & Chabrière, E. (2017). Effect of quorum quenching lactonase in clinical isolates of *Pseudomonas aeruginosa* and comparison with *quorum sensing* inhibitors. *Frontiers in Microbiology, 8*(FEB). https://doi.org/10.3389/fmicb.2017.00227

Gupta, R. K., Luong, T. T., & Lee, C. Y. (2015). RNAIII of the *Staphylococcus aureus agr* system activates global regulator MgrA by stabilizing mRNA. *Proceedings of the National Academy of Sciences of the United States of America, 112*(45). https://doi.org/10.1073/pnas.1509251112

Haaber, J., Penadés, J. R., & Ingmer, H. (2017). Transfer of Antibiotic Resistance in *Staphylococcus aureus. Trends in Microbiology, 25*(11), 893–905. https://doi.org/10.1016/j.tim.2017.05.011

Hammond, E. N., Donkor, E. S., & Brown, C. A. (2014). Biofilm formation of *Clostridium difficile* and susceptibility to Manuka Honey. *BMC Complementary and Alternative Medicine, 14*(1). https://doi.org/10.1186/1472-6882-14-329

Harkins, C. P., Pichon, B., Doumith, M., Parkhill, J., Westh, H., Tomasz, A., de Lencastre, H., Bentley, S. D., Kearns, A. M., & Holden, M. T. G. (2017). Methicillin-resistant *Staphylococcus aureus* emerged long before the introduction of methicillin into clinical practice. *Genome Biology, 18*(1), 1–11. https://doi.org/10.1186/s13059-017-1252-9

Hathroubi, S., Mekni, M. A., Domenico, P., Nguyen, D., & Jacques, M. (2017). Biofilms: Microbial Shelters Against Antibiotics. In *Microbial Drug Resistance* (Vol. 23, Issue 2). https://doi.org/10.1089/mdr.2016.0087

Hatzenbuehler, J., & Pulling, T. J. (2011). Diagnosis and management of osteomyelitis. *American Family Physician*, *84*(9). https://doi.org/10.2165/00019053-199916060-00003

He, L., Le, K. Y., Khan, B. A., Nguyen, T. H., Hunt, R. L., Bae, J. S., Kabat, J., Zheng, Y., Cheung, G. Y. C., Li, M., & Otto, M. (2019). Resistance to leukocytes ties benefits of *quorum sensing* dysfunctionality to biofilm infection. In *Nature Microbiology* (Vol. 4, Issue 7). https://doi.org/10.1038/s41564-019-0413-x

Hemmati, F., Salehi, R., Ghotaslou, R., Kafil, H. S., Hasani, A., Gholizadeh, P., Nouri, R., & Rezaee, M. A. (2020). Quorum quenching: A potential target for antipseudomonal therapy. *Infection and Drug Resistance*, *13*, 2989–3005. https://doi.org/10.2147/IDR.S263196

Hobley, L., Harkins, C., MacPhee, C. E., & Stanley-Wall, N. R. (2015). Giving structure to the biofilm matrix: An overview of individual strategies and emerging common themes. In *FEMS Microbiology Reviews* (Vol. 39, Issue 5). https://doi.org/10.1093/femsre/fuv015

Høyland-Kroghsbo, N. M., Paczkowski, J., Mukherjee, S., Broniewski, J., Westra, E., Bondy-Denomy, J., & Bassler, B. L. (2017). *Quorum sensing* controls the *Pseudomonas aeruginosa* CRISPR-Cas adaptive immune system. *Proceedings of the National Academy of Sciences of the United States of America*, *114*(1). https://doi.org/10.1073/pnas.1617415113

Inoue, Y., Togashi, N., & Hamashima, H. (2016). Farnesol-induced disruption of the *Staphylococcus aureus* cytoplasmic membrane. *Biological and Pharmaceutical Bulletin*, *39*(5). https://doi.org/10.1248/bpb.b15-00416

Ivanova, K., Fernandes, M. M., Mendoza, E., & Tzanov, T. (2015). Enzyme multilayer coatings inhibit *Pseudomonas aeruginosa* biofilm formation on urinary catheters. *Applied Microbiology and Biotechnology*, *99*(10). https://doi.org/10.1007/s00253-015-6378-7

Jenul, C., & Horswill, A. R. (2019). Regulation of *Staphylococcus aureus* Virulence. *Microbiology Spectrum*, *7*(2). https://doi.org/10.1128/microbiolspec.gpp3-0031-2018

Jiang, Q., Chen, J., Yang, C., Yin, Y., Yao, K., & Song, D. (2019). *Quorum Sensing*: A Prospective Therapeutic Target for Bacterial Diseases. *BioMed Research International*, *2019*. https://doi.org/10.1155/2019/2015978

Jiang, Y., Geng, M., & Bai, L. (2020). Targeting biofilms therapy: Current research strategies and development hurdles. *Microorganisms*, *8*(8), 1–34. https://doi.org/10.3390/microorganisms8081222

Jønsson, R., Struve, C., Jenssen, H., & Krogfelt, K. A. (2017). The wax moth *Galleria mellonella* as a novel model system to study Enteroaggregative Escherichia coli pathogenesis. In *Virulence* (Vol. 8, Issue 8). https://doi.org/10.1080/21505594.2016.1256537

Jorjão, A. L., Oliveira, L. D., Scorzoni, L., Figueiredo-Godoi, L. M. A., Prata, M. C. A., Jorge, A. O. C., & Junqueira, J. C. (2018). From moths to caterpillars: Ideal conditions for *Galleria mellonella* rearing for *in vivo* microbiological studies. *Virulence, 9*(1). https://doi.org/10.1080/21505594.2017.1397871

Kalia, V. C. (2013). *Quorum sensing* inhibitors: An overview. In *Biotechnology Advances* (Vol. 31, Issue 2). https://doi.org/10.1016/j.biotechadv.2012.10.004

Kanwar, I., Sah, A. K., & Suresh, P. K. (2017). Biofilm-mediated Antibiotic-resistant Oral Bacterial Infections: Mechanism and Combat Strategies. *Current Pharmaceutical Design, 23*(14). https://doi.org/10.2174/1381612822666161124154549

Karimi, A., Karig, D., Kumar, A., & Ardekani, A. M. (2015). Interplay of physical mechanisms and biofilm processes: Review of microfluidic methods. In *Lab on a Chip* (Vol. 15, Issue 1). https://doi.org/10.1039/c4lc01095g

Ke, M. R., Eastel, J. M., Ngai, K. L. K., Cheung, Y. Y., Chan, P. K. S., Hui, M., Ng, D. K. P., & Lo, P. C. (2014). Photodynamic inactivation of bacteria and viruses using two monosubstituted zinc (II) phthalocyanines. *European Journal of Medicinal Chemistry, 84*. https://doi.org/10.1016/j.ejmech.2014.07.022

Keelara, S., Thakur, S., & Patel, J. (2016). Biofilm formation by environmental isolates of *Salmonella* and their sensitivity to natural antimicrobials. *Foodborne Pathogens and Disease, 13*(9). https://doi.org/10.1089/fpd.2016.2145

Khajanchi, B. K., Kirtley, M. L., Brackman, S. M., & Chopra, A. K. (2011). Immunomodulatory and protective Roles of *quorum-sensing* signaling molecules N-Acyl homoserine lactones during infection of mice with *Aeromonas hydrophila*. *Infection and Immunity, 79*(7). https://doi.org/10.1128/IAI.00096-11

Kim, C., Hesek, D., Lee, M., & Mobashery, S. (2018). Potentiation of the activity of β-lactam antibiotics by farnesol and its derivatives. *Bioorganic and Medicinal Chemistry Letters, 28*(4), 642–645. https://doi.org/10.1016/j.bmcl.2018.01.028

Kolar, S. L., Antonio Ibarra, J., Rivera, F. E., Mootz, J. M., Davenport, J. E., Stevens, S. M., Horswill, A. R., & Shaw, L. N. (2013). Extracellular proteases are key mediators of

Staphylococcus aureus virulence via the global modulation of virulence-determinant stability. *MicrobiologyOpen*, 2(1). https://doi.org/10.1002/mbo3.55

Kothari, V., Sharma, S., & Padia, D. (2017). Recent research advances on *Chromobacterium violaceum*. *Asian Pacific Journal of Tropical Medicine*, 10(8), 744–752. https://doi.org/10.1016/j.apjtm.2017.07.022

Koul, S., Prakash, J., Mishra, A., & Kalia, V. C. (2016). Potential Emergence of Multi-*quorum sensing* Inhibitor Resistant (MQSIR) Bacteria. In *Indian Journal of Microbiology* (Vol. 56, Issue 1). https://doi.org/10.1007/s12088-015-0558-0

Krol, E., & Becker, A. (2014). Rhizobial homologs of the fatty acid transporter FadL facilitate perception of long-chain acyl-homoserine lactone signals. *Proceedings of the National Academy of Sciences of the United States of America*, 111(29). https://doi.org/10.1073/pnas.1404929111

LaSarre, B., & Federle, M. J. (2013). Exploiting *Quorum Sensing* to Confuse Bacterial Pathogens. *Microbiology and Molecular Biology Reviews*, 77(1). https://doi.org/10.1128/mmbr.00046-12

Le, K. Y., & Otto, M. (2015). *Quorum-sensing* regulation in staphylococci-an overview. *Frontiers in Microbiology*, 6(OCT), 1–8. https://doi.org/10.3389/fmicb.2015.01174

Lee, J., Wu, J., Deng, Y., Wang, J., Wang, C., Wang, J., Chang, C., Dong, Y., Williams, P., & Zhang, L. H. (2013). A cell-cell communication signal integrates quorum sensing and stress response. *Nature Chemical Biology*, 9(5). https://doi.org/10.1038/nchembio.1225

Lee, J., & Zhang, L. (2014). The hierarchy *quorum sensing* network in *Pseudomonas aeruginosa*. *Protein and Cell*, 6(1). https://doi.org/10.1007/s13238-014-0100-x

Li, S., Chen, S., Fan, J., Cao, Z., Ouyang, W., Tong, N., Hu, X., Hu, J., Li, P., Feng, Z., Huang, X., Li, Y., Xie, M., He, R., Jian, J., Wu, B., Xu, C., Wu, W., Guo, J., Sun, P. (2018). Anti-biofilm effect of novel thiazole acid analogs against *Pseudomonas aeruginosa* through IQS pathways. *European Journal of Medicinal Chemistry*, 145. https://doi.org/10.1016/j.ejmech.2017.12.076

Li, Y., Xiao, P., Wang, Y., & Hao, Y. (2020). Mechanisms and Control Measures of Mature Biofilm Resistance to Antimicrobial Agents in the Clinical Context. *ACS Omega*. https://doi.org/10.1021/acsomega.0c02294

Lin, M. F., Lin, Y. Y., Tu, C. C., & Lan, C. Y. (2017). Distribution of different efflux pump genes in clinical isolates of multidrug-resistant *Acinetobacter baumannii* and their correlation with antimicrobial resistance. *Journal of Microbiology, Immunology and Infection*, *50*(2). https://doi.org/10.1016/j.jmii.2015.04.004

Linnes, J. C., Ma, H., & Bryers, J. D. (2013). Giant extracellular matrix binding protein expression in *Staphylococcus epidermidis* is regulated by biofilm formation and osmotic pressure. *Current Microbiology*, *66*(6). https://doi.org/10.1007/s00284-013-0316-7

Little, B. J., & Lee, J. S. (2014). Microbiologically influenced corrosion: An update. In *International Materials Reviews* (Vol. 59, Issue 7). https://doi.org/10.1179/1743280414Y.0000000035

Liu, W., Ran, C., Liu, Z., Gao, Q., Xu, S., Ringø, E., Myklebust, R., Gu, Z., & Zhou, Z. (2016). Effects of dietary *Lactobacillus plantarum* and AHL lactonase on the control of *Aeromonas hydrophila* infection in tilapia. *Microbiology Open*, *5*(4). https://doi.org/10.1002/mbo3.362

Liu, Y. C., Chan, K. G., & Chang, C. Y. (2015). Modulation of host biology by *Pseudomonas aeruginosa quorum sensing* signal molecules: Messengers or traitors. In *Frontiers in Microbiology* (Vol. 6, Issue NOV). https://doi.org/10.3389/fmicb.2015.01226

Liu, Y., Mu, C., Ying, X., Li, W., Wu, N., Dong, J., Gao, Y., Shao, N., Fan, M., & Yang, G. (2011). RNAIII activates *map* expression by forming an RNA-RNA complex in *Staphylococcus aureus. FEBS Letters*, *585*(6). https://doi.org/10.1016/j.febslet.2011.02.021

Lozano, C., Azcona-Gutiérrez, J. M., van Bambeke, F., & Sáenz, Y. (2018). Great phenotypic and genetic variation among successive chronic *Pseudomonas aeruginosa* from a cystic fibrosis patient. *PLoS ONE*, *13*(9). https://doi.org/10.1371/journal.pone.0204167

Madsen, J. S., Burmølle, M., Hansen, L. H., & Sørensen, S. J. (2012). The interconnection between biofilm formation and horizontal gene transfer. In *FEMS Immunology and Medical Microbiology* (Vol. 65, Issue 2). https://doi.org/10.1111/j.1574-695X.2012.00960.x

Mah, T. F. (2012). Biofilm-specific antibiotic resistance. In *Future Microbiology* (Vol. 7, Issue 9). https://doi.org/10.2217/fmb.12.76

Maisonneuve, E., & Gerdes, K. (2014). Molecular mechanisms underlying bacterial persisters. In *Cell* (Vol. 157, Issue 3). https://doi.org/10.1016/j.cell.2014.02.050

Malhotra, S., Hayes, D., & Wozniak, D. J. (2019). Cystic fibrosis and *Pseudomonas aeruginosa*: The host-microbe interface. In *Clinical Microbiology Reviews* (Vol. 32, Issue 3). https://doi.org/10.1128/CMR.00138-18

Martinez, J. L. (2014). General principles of antibiotic resistance in bacteria. *Drug Discovery Today: Technologies*, *11*(1), 33–39. https://doi.org/10.1016/j.ddtec.2014.02.001

Mathias, J., & Stoodley, P. (2011). Biofilm Highlights. *Advances*, *5*. https://doi.org/10.1007/978-3-642-19940-0

McBrayer, D. N., Cameron, C. D., & Tal-Gan, Y. (2020). Development and utilization of peptide-based *quorum sensing* modulators in Gram-positive bacteria. *Organic & Biomolecular Chemistry*, *18*(37), 7273–7290. https://doi.org/10.1039/d0ob01421d

Mellbye, B., & Schuster, M. (2011). The sociomicrobiology of antivirulence drug resistance: A proof of concept. *MBio*, *2*(5). https://doi.org/10.1128/mBio.00131-11

Mok, N., Chan, S. Y., Liu, S. Y., & Chua, S. L. (2020). Vanillin inhibits PqsR-mediated virulence in *Pseudomonas aeruginosa*. *Food & Function*, *11*(7), 6496–6508. https://doi.org/10.1039/d0fo00046a

Monnet, V., & Gardan, R. (2015). *Quorum-sensing* regulators in Gram-positive bacteria: "cherchez le peptide." In *Molecular Microbiology* (Vol. 97, Issue 2). https://doi.org/10.1111/mmi.13060

Montgomery, C. P., Boyle-Vavra, S., Roux, A., Ebine, K., Sonenshein, A. L., & Daumb, R. S. (2012). CodY deletion enhances in vivo virulence of community-associated methicillin-resistant *Staphylococcus aureus* clone USA300. *Infection and Immunity*, *80*(7), 2382–2389. https://doi.org/10.1128/IAI.06172-11

Moons, P., Michiels, C. W., & Aertsen, A. (2009). Bacterial interactions in biofilms. *Critical Reviews in Microbiology*, *35*(3), 157–168. https://doi.org/10.1080/10408410902809431

Moreau, P., Diggle, S. P., & Friman, V. P. (2017). Bacterial cell-to-cell signaling promotes the evolution of resistance to parasitic bacteriophages. *Ecology and Evolution*, *7*(6). https://doi.org/10.1002/ece3.2818

Morrison, J. M., Anderson, K. L., Beenken, K. E., Smeltzer, M. S., & Dunman, P. M. (2012). The *staphylococcal* accessory regulator, SarA, is an RNA-binding protein that modulates the mRNA turnover properties of late-exponential and stationary phase *Staphylococcus aureus* cells. *Frontiers in Cellular and Infection Microbiology*, *2*. https://doi.org/10.3389/fcimb.2012.00026

Mukherjee, S., & Bassler, B. L. (2019). Bacterial *quorum sensing* in complex and dynamically changing environments. *Nature Reviews Microbiology*, *17*(6), 371–382. https://doi.org/10.1038/s41579-019-0186-5

Mukherjee, S., Moustafa, D. A., Stergioula, V., Smith, C. D., Goldberg, J. B., & Bassler, B. L. (2018). The PqsE and RhlR proteins are an autoinducer synthase–receptor pair that control virulence and biofilm development in *Pseudomonas aeruginosa*. *Proceedings of the National Academy of Sciences of the United States of America*, *115*(40). https://doi.org/10.1073/pnas.1814023115

Neu, T. R., & Lawrence, J. R. (2014). Advanced techniques for in situ analysis of the biofilm matrix (Structure, Composition, Dynamics) by means of laser scanning microscopy. *Methods in Molecular Biology*, *1147*. https://doi.org/10.1007/978-1-4939-0467-9_4

Ng, W. L., & Bassler, B. L. (2009). Bacterial *quorum-sensing* network architectures. In *Annual Review of Genetics* (Vol. 43). https://doi.org/10.1146/annurev-genet-102108-134304

O'Loughlin, C. T., Miller, L. C., Siryaporn, A., Drescher, K., Semmelhack, M. F., & Bassler, B. L. (2013). A *quorum-sensing* inhibitor blocks *Pseudomonas aeruginosa* virulence and biofilm formation. *Proceedings of the National Academy of Sciences of the United States of America*, *110*(44). https://doi.org/10.1073/pnas.1316981110

Olsen, I. (2015). Biofilm-specific antibiotic tolerance and resistance. In *European Journal of Clinical Microbiology and Infectious Diseases* (Vol. 34, Issue 5). https://doi.org/10.1007/s10096-015-2323-z

Omidi, M., Firoozeh, F., Saffari, M., Sedaghat, H., Zibaei, M., & Khaledi, A. (2020). Ability of biofilm production and molecular analysis of *spa* and *ica* genes among clinical isolates of methicillin-resistant *Staphylococcus aureus*. *BMC Research Notes*, *13*(1), 1–7. https://doi.org/10.1186/s13104-020-4885-9

O'Neill, J. (2016). Tackling drug-resistant infections globally: final report and recommendations the review on antimicrobial resistance. Review on Antimicrobial Resistance, https://amr-review.org/sites/default/files/160525_Final%20paper_with%20cover.pdf

Otto, M. (2004). *Quorum-sensing* control in *Staphylococci* - A target for antimicrobial drug therapy? *FEMS Microbiology Letters*, *241*(2), 135–141. https://doi.org/10.1016/j.femsle.2004.11.016

Otto, M. (2013). *Staphylococcal* infections: Mechanisms of biofilm maturation and detachment as critical determinants of pathogenicity. *Annual Review of Medicine*, *64*. https://doi.org/10.1146/annurev-med-042711-140023

Paczkowski, J. E., Mukherjee, S., McCready, A. R., Cong, J. P., Aquino, C. J., Kim, H., Henke, B. R., Smith, C. D., & Bassler, B. L. (2017). Flavonoids suppress *Pseudomonas aeruginosa* virulence through allosteric inhibition of *quorum-sensing* Receptors. *Journal of Biological Chemistry*, *292*(10). https://doi.org/10.1074/jbc.M116.770552

Palliyil, S., Downham, C., Broadbent, I., Charlton, K., & Porter, A. J. (2014). High-Sensitivity Monoclonal Antibodies Specific for Homoserine Lactones Protect Mice from Lethal *Pseudomonas aeruginosa* Infections. *Applied and Environmental Microbiology*, *80*(2). https://doi.org/10.1128/AEM.02912-13

Papenfort, K., & Bassler, B. L. (2016). *Quorum sensing* signal-response systems in Gram-negative bacteria. *Nature Reviews Microbiology*, *14*(9), 576–588. https://doi.org/10.1038/nrmicro.2016.89

Pérez-Pérez, M., Jorge, P., Pérez Rodríguez, G., Pereira, M. O., & Lourenço, A. (2017). *Quorum sensing* inhibition in *Pseudomonas aeruginosa* biofilms: new insights through network mining. *Biofouling*, *33*(2), 128–142. https://doi.org/10.1080/08927014.2016.1272104

Petrova, O. E., & Sauer, K. (2016). Escaping the biofilm in more than one way: Desorption, detachment or dispersion. In *Current Opinion in Microbiology* (Vol. 30). https://doi.org/10.1016/j.mib.2016.01.004

Pontes, D. S., de Araujo, R. S. A., Dantas, N., Scotti, L., Scotti, M. T., de Moura, R. O., & Mendonca-Junior, F. J. B. (2018). Genetic Mechanisms of Antibiotic Resistance and the Role of Antibiotic Adjuvants. *Current Topics in Medicinal Chemistry*, *18*(1), 42–74. https://doi.org/10.2174/1568026618666180206095224

Popp, P. F., & Mascher, T. (2019). Coordinated Cell Death in Isogenic Bacterial Populations: Sacrificing Some for the Benefit of Many? In *Journal of Molecular Biology* (Vol. 431, Issue 23). https://doi.org/10.1016/j.jmb.2019.04.024

Priyadarshi, A., Kim, E. E., & Hwang, K. Y. (2010). Structural insights into *Staphylococcus aureus* enoyl-ACP reductase (FabI), in complex with NADP end triclosan. *Proteins: Structure, Function and Bioinformatics*, *78*(2). https://doi.org/10.1002/prot.22581

Pustelny, C., Albers, A., Büldt-Karentzopoulos, K., Parschat, K., Chhabra, S. R., Cámara, M., Williams, P., & Fetzner, S. (2009). Dioxygenase-Mediated Quenching of Quinolone-Dependent *Quorum Sensing* in *Pseudomonas aeruginosa*. *Chemistry and Biology, 16*(12). https://doi.org/10.1016/j.chembiol.2009.11.013

Rajasree, K., Fasim, A., & Gopal, B. (2016). Conformational features of the *Staphylococcus aureus* AgrA-promoter interactions rationalize *quorum-sensing* triggered gene expression. *Biochemistry and Biophysics Reports, 6*. https://doi.org/10.1016/j.bbrep.2016.03.012

Romaní, A. M., Fund, K., Artigas, J., Schwartz, T., Sabater, S., & Obst, U. (2008). Relevance of polymeric matrix enzymes during biofilm formation. *Microbial Ecology, 56*(3). https://doi.org/10.1007/s00248-007-9361-8

Rossiter, S. E., Fletcher, M. H., & Wuest, W. M. (2017). Natural Products as Platforms to Overcome Antibiotic Resistance. *Chemical Reviews, 117*(19), 12415–12474. https://doi.org/10.1021/acs.chemrev.7b00283

Roux, A., Todd, D. A., Velázquez, J. v., Cech, N. B., & Sonenshein, A. L. (2014). CodY-Mediated regulation of the *Staphylococcus aureus* Agr System integrates nutritional and population density signals. *Journal of Bacteriology, 196*(6). https://doi.org/10.1128/JB.00128-13

Roy, R., Tiwari, M., Donelli, G., & Tiwari, V. (2018). Strategies for combating bacterial biofilms: A focus on anti-biofilm agents and their mechanisms of action. *Virulence, 9*(1), 522–554. https://doi.org/10.1080/21505594.2017.1313372

Rutherford, S. T., & Bassler, B. L. (2012). Bacterial *quorum sensing*: Its role in virulence and possibilities for its control. *Cold Spring Harbor Perspectives in Medicine, 2*(11), 1–25. https://doi.org/10.1101/cshperspect.a012427

Sakr, M. M., Aboshanab, K. M., Elkhatib, W. F., Yassien, M. A., & Hassouna, N. A. (2018). Overexpressed recombinant quorum quenching lactonase reduces the virulence, motility and biofilm formation of multidrug-resistant *Pseudomonas aeruginosa* clinical isolates. *Applied Microbiology and Biotechnology, 102*(24). https://doi.org/10.1007/s00253-018-9418-2

Sankar Ganesh, P., & Ravishankar Rai, V. (2018). Attenuation of *quorum-sensing*-dependent virulence factors and biofilm formation by medicinal plants against antibiotic resistant *Pseudomonas aeruginosa*. *Journal of Traditional and Complementary Medicine, 8*(1). https://doi.org/10.1016/j.jtcme.2017.05.008

Saville, R. M., Rakshe, S., Haagensen, J. A. J., Shukla, S., & Spormann, A. M. (2011). Energy-dependent stability of *Shewanella oneidensis* MR-1 biofilms. *Journal of Bacteriology, 193*(13). https://doi.org/10.1128/JB.00251-11

Saxena, P., Joshi, Y., Rawat, K., & Bisht, R. (2019). Biofilms: Architecture, Resistance, *Quorum Sensing* and Control Mechanisms. In *Indian Journal of Microbiology* (Vol. 59, Issue 1). https://doi.org/10.1007/s12088-018-0757-6

Schertzer, J. W., Brown, S. A., & Whiteley, M. (2010). Oxygen levels rapidly modulate *Pseudomonas aeruginosa* social behaviours via substrate limitation of PqsH. *Molecular Microbiology, 77*(6). https://doi.org/10.1111/j.1365-2958.2010.07303.x

Schuster, M., Sexton1, D. J., & Hense, B. A. (2017). Why *quorum sensing* controls private goods. *Frontiers in Microbiology, 8*(MAY). https://doi.org/10.3389/fmicb.2017.00885

Sebaa, S., Hizette, N., Boucherit-Otmani, Z., & Courtois, P. (2017). Dose-dependent effect of lysozyme upon *Candida albicans* biofilm. *Molecular Medicine Reports, 15*(3). https://doi.org/10.3892/mmr.2017.6148

Serra, D. O., Richter, A. M., & Hengge, R. (2013). Cellulose as an architectural element in spatially structured *Escherichia coli* biofilms. *Journal of Bacteriology, 195*(24). https://doi.org/10.1128/JB.00946-13

Silva, L. N., da Hora, G. C. A., Soares, T. A., Bojer, M. S., Ingmer, H., Macedo, A. J., & Trentin, D. S. (2017). Myricetin protects *Galleria mellonella* against *Staphylococcus aureus* infection and inhibits multiple virulence factors. *Scientific Reports, 7*(1), 1–16. https://doi.org/10.1038/s41598-017-02712-1

Sloan, T. J., Murray, E., Yokoyama, M., Massey, R. C., Chan, W. C., Bonev, B. B., & Williams, P. (2019). Timing is everything: Impact of naturally occurring *Staphylococcus aureus* AgrC cytoplasmic domain adaptive mutations on autoinduction. *Journal of Bacteriology, 201*(20). https://doi.org/10.1128/JB.00409-19

Soh, E. Y. C., Chhabra, S. R., Halliday, N., Heeb, S., Müller, C., Birmes, F. S., Fetzner, S., Cámara, M., Chan, K. G., & Williams, P. (2015). Biotic inactivation of the *Pseudomonas aeruginosa* quinolone signal molecule. *Environmental Microbiology, 17*(11). https://doi.org/10.1111/1462-2920.12857

Starkey, M., Lepine, F., Maura, D., Bandyopadhaya, A., Lesic, B., He, J., Kitao, T., Righi, V., Milot, S., Tzika, A., & Rahme, L. (2014). Identification of Anti-virulence Compounds

That Disrupt *Quorum-Sensing* Regulated Acute and Persistent Pathogenicity. *PLoS Pathogens*, *10*(8). https://doi.org/10.1371/journal.ppat.1004321

Stepanović, S., Vuković, D., Hola, V., Bonaventura, G. di, Djukić, S., Ćircović, I., & Ruzicka, F. (2007). Quantification of biofilm in microtiter plates. *Apmis*, *115*(8), 891–899.

Stoodley, P., Sauer, K., Davies, D. G., & Costerton, J. W. (2002). Biofilms as complex differentiated communities. In *Annual Review of Microbiology* (Vol. 56). https://doi.org/10.1146/annurev.micro.56.012302.160705

Sun, S., Zhou, L., Jin, K., Jiang, H., & He, Y. W. (2016). *Quorum sensing* systems differentially regulate the production of phenazine-1-carboxylic acid in the rhizobacterium *Pseudomonas aeruginosa* PA1201. *Scientific Reports*, *6*. https://doi.org/10.1038/srep30352

Tan, L., Li, S. R., Jiang, B., Hu, X. M., & Li, S. (2018). Therapeutic targeting of the *Staphylococcus aureus* accessory gene regulator (*agr*) system. *Frontiers in Microbiology*, *9*(JAN), 1–11. https://doi.org/10.3389/fmicb.2018.00055

Taszłow, P., Vertyporokh, L., & Wojda, I. (2017). Humoral immune response of *Galleria mellonella* after repeated infection with *Bacillus thuringiensis. Journal of Invertebrate Pathology*, *149*(July), 87–96. https://doi.org/10.1016/j.jip.2017.08.008

Thoendel, M., Kavanaugh, J. S., Flack, C. E., & Horswill, A. R. (2011). Peptide signaling in the *Staphylococci. Chemical Reviews*, *111*(1). https://doi.org/10.1021/cr100370n

Tielen, P., Kuhn, H., Rosenau, F., Jaeger, K. E., Flemming, H. C., & Wingender, J. (2013). Interaction between extracellular lipase LipA and the polysaccharide alginate of *Pseudomonas aeruginosa. BMC Microbiology*, *13*(1). https://doi.org/10.1186/1471-2180-13-159

Tomioka, H., Sano, C., & Tatano, Y. (2017). Host-Directed Therapeutics against Mycobacterial Infections. *Current Pharmaceutical Design*, *23*(18). https://doi.org/10.2174/1381612822666161202121550

Tsai, C. J. Y., Loh, J. M. S., & Proft, T. (2016). *Galleria mellonella* infection models for the study of bacterial diseases and for antimicrobial drug testing. *Virulence*, *7*(3), 214–229. https://doi.org/10.1080/21505594.2015.1135289

Tsai, T., Chien, H. F., Wang, T. H., Huang, C. T., Ker, Y. B., & Chen, C. T. (2011). Chitosan augments photodynamic inactivation of gram-positive and gram-negative bacteria. *Antimicrobial Agents and Chemotherapy*, *55*(5). https://doi.org/10.1128/AAC.00550-10

Turan, N. B., Chormey, D. S., Büyükpınar, Ç., Engin, G. O., & Bakirdere, S. (2017). *Quorum sensing*: Little talks for an effective bacterial coordination. In *TrAC - Trends in Analytical Chemistry* (Vol. 91). https://doi.org/10.1016/j.trac.2017.03.007

U.S Department of Health and Human Services. (2019). Antibiotic resistance threats in the United States. *Centers for Disease Control and Prevention*, 1–113. https://www.cdc.gov/drugresistance/biggest_threats.html

Vadekeetil, A., Saini, H., Chhibber, S., & Harjai, K. (2016). Exploiting the antivirulence efficacy of an ajoene-ciprofloxacin combination against *Pseudomonas aeruginosa* biofilm associated murine acute pyelonephritis. *Biofouling*, *32*(4). https://doi.org/10.1080/08927014.2015.1137289

Vert, M., Doi, Y., Hellwich, K. H., Hess, M., Hodge, P., Kubisa, P., Rinaudo, M., & Schué, F. (2012). Terminology for biorelated polymers and applications (IUPAC recommendations 2012). *Pure and Applied Chemistry*, *84*(2). https://doi.org/10.1351/pac-rec-10-12-04

Waglechner, N., & Wright, G. D. (2017). Antibiotic resistance: It's bad, but why isn't it worse? *BMC Biology*, *15*(1), 1–8. https://doi.org/10.1186/s12915-017-0423-1

Wang, R., Khan, B. A., Cheung, G. Y. C., Bach, T. H. L., Jameson-Lee, M., Kong, K. F., Queck, S. Y., & Otto, M. (2011). *Staphylococcus epidermidis* surfactant peptides promote biofilm maturation and dissemination of biofilm-associated infection in mice. *Journal of Clinical Investigation*, *121*(1). https://doi.org/10.1172/JCI42520

Weaver, L., Webber, J. B., Hickson, A. C., Abraham, P. M., & Close, M. E. (2015). Biofilm resilience to desiccation in groundwater aquifers: A laboratory and field study. *Science of the Total Environment*, *514*. https://doi.org/10.1016/j.scitotenv.2014.10.031

Welsh, M. A., & Blackwell, H. E. (2016). Chemical Genetics Reveals Environment-Specific Roles for *Quorum Sensing* Circuits in *Pseudomonas aeruginosa*. *Cell Chemical Biology*, *23*(3). https://doi.org/10.1016/j.chembiol.2016.01.006

Weng, L. X., Yang, Y. X., Zhang, Y. Q., & Wang, L. H. (2014). A new synthetic ligand that activates QscR and blocks antibiotic-tolerant biofilm formation in *Pseudomonas aeruginosa*. *Applied Microbiology and Biotechnology*, *98*(6). https://doi.org/10.1007/s00253-013-5420-x

Whitfield, G. B., Marmont, L. S., & Howell, P. L. (2015). Enzymatic modifications of exopolysaccharides enhance bacterial persistence. In *Frontiers in Microbiology* (Vol. 6, Issue MAY). https://doi.org/10.3389/fmicb.2015.00596

World Health Organization (2015). Global Action Plan on Antimicrobial Resistance. *Microbe Magazine, 10*(9), 354–355. https://doi.org/10.1128/microbe.10.354.1

World Health Organization (2017). A European One Health Action Plan against Antimicrobial Resistance (AMR). *European Commission, Last visit,* 24. http://www.who.int/entity/drugresistance/documents/surveillancereport/en/index.html%0Ahttp://www.who.int/entity/drugresistance/documents/surveillancereport/en/index.html%250Ahttp://www.who.int/entity/drugresistance/documents/surveillancereport/en/index.ht

World Health Organization (2017). Global priority list of antibiotic-resistant bacteria to guide research, discovery, and development of new antibiotics. https://www.who.int/medicines/publications/global-priority-list-antibiotic-resistant-bacteria/en/

Wilde, A. D., Snyder, D. J., Putnam, N. E., Valentino, M. D., Hammer, N. D., Lonergan, Z. R., Hinger, S. A., Aysanoa, E. E., Blanchard, C., Dunman, P. M., Wasserman, G. A., Chen, J., Shopsin, B., Gilmore, M. S., Skaar, E. P., & Cassat, J. E. (2015). Bacterial Hypoxic Responses Revealed as Critical Determinants of the Host-Pathogen Outcome by TnSeq Analysis of *Staphylococcus aureus* Invasive Infection. *PLoS Pathogens, 11*(12). https://doi.org/10.1371/journal.ppat.1005341

Wilking, J. N., Zaburdaev, V., de Volder, M., Losick, R., Brenner, M. P., & Weitz, D. A. (2013). Liquid transport facilitated by channels in *Bacillus subtilis* biofilms. *Proceedings of the National Academy of Sciences of the United States of America, 110*(3). https://doi.org/10.1073/pnas.1216376110

Wingender, J., & Flemming, H. C. (2011). Biofilms in drinking water and their role as reservoir for pathogens. *International Journal of Hygiene and Environmental Health, 214*(6). https://doi.org/10.1016/j.ijheh.2011.05.009

Yadav, M. K., Park, S. W., Chae, S. W., & Song, J. J. (2014). Sinefungin, a natural nucleoside analogue of S-adenosylmethionine, inhibits *Streptococcus pneumoniae* biofilm growth. *BioMed Research International, 2014.* https://doi.org/10.1155/2014/156987

Yan, J., & Bassler, B. L. (2019). Surviving as a Community: Antibiotic Tolerance and Persistence in Bacterial Biofilms. *Cell Host and Microbe, 26*(1), 15–21. https://doi.org/10.1016/j.chom.2019.06.002

Yang, Y. X., Xu, Z. H., Zhang, Y. Q., Tian, J., Weng, L. X., & Wang, L. H. (2012). A new *quorum-sensing* inhibitor attenuates virulence and decreases antibiotic resistance in *Pseudomonas aeruginosa*. *Journal of Microbiology*, *50*(6). https://doi.org/10.1007/s12275-012-2149-7

Zelezniak, A., Andrejev, S., Ponomarova, O., Mende, D. R., Bork, P., & Patil, K. R. (2015). Metabolic dependencies drive species co-occurrence in diverse microbial communities. *Proceedings of the National Academy of Sciences of the United States of America*, *112*(20). https://doi.org/10.1073/pnas.1421834112

Zhang, Weipeng, Sun, J., Ding, W., Lin, J., Tian, R., Lu, L., Liu, X., Shen, X., & Qian, P. Y. (2015). Extracellular matrix-associated proteins form an integral and dynamic system during *Pseudomonas aeruginosa* biofilm development. *Frontiers in Cellular and Infection Microbiology*, *5*(MAY). https://doi.org/10.3389/fcimb.2015.00040

Zhang, Weiwei, & Li, C. (2016). Exploiting *quorum sensing* interfering strategies in gram-negative bacteria for the enhancement of environmental applications. *Frontiers in Microbiology*, *6*(JAN). https://doi.org/10.3389/fmicb.2015.01535

Zhang, X., Ou-yang, S., Wang, J., Liao, L., Wu, R., & Wei, J. (2018). Construction of Antibacterial Surface via Layer-by-Layer Method. *Current Pharmaceutical Design*, *24*. https://doi.org/10.2174/1381612824666180219125655

Zhao, X., Yu, Z., & Ding, T. (2020). *Quorum-sensing* regulation of antimicrobial resistance in bacteria. *Microorganisms*, *8*(3), 1–21. https://doi.org/10.3390/microorganisms8030425

Zielinska, A. K., Beenken, K. E., Joo, H. S., Mrak, L. N., Griffin, L. M., Luong, T. T., Lee, C. Y., Otto, M., Shaw, L. N., & Smeltzer, M. S. (2011). Defining the strain-dependent impact of the *staphylococcal* accessory regulator (sarA) on the alpha-toxin phenotype of *Staphylococcus aureus*. *Journal of Bacteriology*, *193*(12). https://doi.org/10.1128/JB.01517-10